T0366202

"Tekin integrates brilliantly the medical humanities, ethics, and the philosophies of science and mind in presenting her compelling vision of what person-centered mental health treatment will look like. A landmark work."

Owen Flanagan Jr., *distinguished professor emeritus of philosophy, Duke University*

"This book is an achievement and a breath of fresh air. Tekin develops a wonderfully readable, deeply informed, and altogether convincing rebuttal of the reductionism that shapes contemporary approaches to the mind. Her project re-humanizes psychiatry by putting the self back where it belongs, at the center of theory and practice."

Dan Kelly, *professor of philosophy, Purdue University*

"Tekin's analysis of the lack of attention to the self and the importance of lived experiences in psychiatry is spot-on. Tekin's MuSe model points the way forward to a scientifically sound, helpful, and ethical psychiatric practice. Must read for practitioners, bioethicists, and philosophers of science alike!"

Kristien Hens, *professor of philosophy, University of Antwerp*

"Tekin combines fascinating case studies of mental illness with deep understanding of psychiatry, psychology, and philosophy. She develops a rich model of the self that contributes greatly to the theory and practice of helping people overcome psychiatric problems. It is a landmark in the philosophy of psychiatry."

Paul Thagard, *distinguished professor emeritus of philosophy, University of Waterloo*

"Tekin's new book restores the practical and clinical importance of the 'self' to mental health research and practice. In these pages, clinicians, investigators, and psychiatric service users will find new pathways to personal and empirical-scientific understandings, while enriching themselves in the process."

John Sadler, *professor of psychiatry, University of Texas Southwestern*

"How patients experience their own condition would seem central to psychiatry, but the self has long been overlooked by a discipline obsessed with establishing its scientific standing. In this beautifully written book, Tekin challenges this neglect and promises to revolutionize psychiatry by foregrounding patients' selves and their testimonies. With this groundbreaking book, psychiatry can at last reclaim subjectivity."

Edouard Machery, *distinguished professor and director of the Center for Philosophy of Science, University of Pittsburgh*

Reclaiming the Self in Psychiatry

Reclaiming the Self in Psychiatry: Centering Personal Narratives for Humanist Science diagnoses the fundamental problem in contemporary scientific psychiatry to be a lack of a sophisticated and nuanced engagement with the self and proposes a solution—the Multitudinous Self Model (*MuSe*).

MuSe fulfils psychiatry's twin commitments to patients' flourishing and scientific objectivity. Marshalling the conceptual and empirical resources from testimonies from individuals diagnosed with mental disorders, substantive research in cognitive science, and empirically informed philosophy, *MuSe* provides clinicians, scientists, and patients pathways to respond to mental distresses and disorders. This framework boosts psychiatry's relationship to science by facilitating expansive notions of expertise and objectivity in which some patients are recognized as "experience-based experts" whose contributions to psychiatric knowledge are indispensable. Şerife Tekin draws the contours of a future for psychiatry that is grounded in philosophy, medical humanities, and social sciences as much as physiology and neuroscience.

This book is an ideal read for professional psychiatrists and philosophers of psychiatry who are interested in the philosophy of mental health.

Şerife Tekin, PhD, is an associate professor at the Center for Bioethics and Humanities at SUNY Upstate Medical University in Syracuse, NY. She co-edited *The Handbook of Psychiatric Ethics* (Oxford University Press, 2021), *The Bloomsbury Companion to Philosophy and Psychiatry* (Bloomsbury, 2019), and *Extraordinary Science and Psychiatry: Responses to the Crisis in Mental Health Research* (MIT Press, 2017). Her articles appeared in *Philosophy of Science; Synthese; American Journal of Bioethics*, and elsewhere.

Reclaiming the Self in Psychiatry

Centering Personal Narratives for a Humanist Science

Şerife Tekin

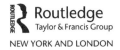
Routledge
Taylor & Francis Group
NEW YORK AND LONDON

Designed cover image: Getty Images © stellalevi

First published 2025
by Routledge
605 Third Avenue, New York, NY 10158

and by Routledge
4 Park Square, Milton Park, Abingdon, Oxon OX14 4RN

Routledge is an imprint of the Taylor & Francis Group, an informa business

© 2025 Şerife Tekin

The right of Şerife Tekin to be identified as author of this work has been asserted in accordance with sections 77 and 78 of the Copyright, Designs and Patents Act 1988.

ISBN: 978-0-367-51813-4 (hbk)
ISBN: 978-0-367-51811-0 (pbk)
ISBN: 978-1-003-05555-6 (ebk)

DOI: 10.4324/9781003055556

Typeset in Sabon
by Taylor & Francis Books

I dedicate this book to my mother, Bahriye Tekin, who, in reclaiming her self, helped her three daughters and their dreams to flourish in a society that has always missed the moment. Without her, I would not be who I am.

Contents

List of Tables

Acknowledgments

Though I didn't realize it at the time, I started writing this book in 2011, during a conversation with Jackie Sullivan after she provided a commentary on a talk I gave at the Southern Society for Philosophy and Psychology (SSPP) meeting in New Orleans. The talk was based on a chapter of my recently defended PhD dissertation, in which I argued that psychiatric diagnoses serve as a source of self-narratives—for better or worse—and that any philosophical investigation of the scientific credibility of psychiatric classifications must take into account the ways in which diagnoses interact with the individuals who are subject to mental disorder diagnoses. Her first response to my talk was to say, "No one talks about the self anymore!" Her acute observation and summary of my project started to shape a research program that eventually led me to write this book. Jackie gave me the words to define my philosophical mission to trace how the self has gone missing and how to best reclaim it, not only in psychiatry, but also in philosophy. I am grateful to Jackie for her commentary and her continued enthusiasm for my work since then.

Words escape me when I try to describe the magnitude of my indebtedness to Dan Kelly. He has generously been sharing his brain with me since I met him back in 2014 at another meeting of the SSPP, in Charleston. He was there when I first started to brainstorm about the book, in its embryonic form. He came to my rescue whenever I was stuck sorting out the messy literature on the self or disarmed by critics who insisted that the self was not worthy of philosophical attention. He carefully read numerous drafts of the book manuscript and gave excellent feedback. He helped me write the book *I* wanted to write and cheered me on even when I was ready to give up. Without him, this book would not have been possible.

I thank the Ann Johnson Institute for Science, Technology, and Society at the University of South Carolina for their generous support, which included holding a book manuscript workshop that enabled me to receive extremely helpful comments from the giants in the field. I am grateful to Leah McClimans, Allison Marsh, Rachel Ankeny, Miriam Solomon, Dan Kelly, George Khushf, Agnes Bolinska, and Riana Betzler for giving me feedback about the draft manuscript. I am also thankful to Rachell Powell, Megan Delehanty, Owen Flanagan, and Frankie Egan for reading the final draft of the book and providing me with valuable comments. I thank Elizabeth Thompson and Sophie Pollack-Milgate for the tremendous research and editorial support they provided for the project.

I am thankful to my early mentors, who introduced me to doing philosophy in North America. The late Ian Hacking supported my strategy to turn to first-person accounts of individuals diagnosed with mental disorders into philosophical contemplation of psychopathology, continuously alleviating my worries about whether or how the method would fly in philosophy. Kristin Andrews introduced me to cognitive science, inspired me to look for empirical grounds to bolster my philosophical claims about the self and mental disorder, and taught me how to ask important questions about scientific methodology. David Jopling infused skepticism into how I do philosophy, which, luckily, still prevents me from falling into dogmatism and reminds me to always turn to the real world to seek answers to philosophical questions. I am also indebted to the students I have mentored as a part of the York University's Center for Students with Dis/abilities mentorship program, who were returning back to school after a period of psychiatric hospitalization; their expertise taught me so much about flourishing.

I was fortunate to have received fellowships and grants that have supported me as I worked on the project. I am grateful for the fellowships I received from the Center for Philosophy of Science, University of Pittsburgh. After providing me with a philosophical home back in 2012–13, when I was hired as Postdoctoral Research Fellow, the Center took me in again, as a Visiting Fellow in 2022. It is during that time I finally had the time and space to start writing the book and finished a first draft. I am also grateful for the fellowships I have received from the Rotman Institute of Philosophy at Western University, and the Lutcher Brown Distinguished Faculty Program at the University of Texas at San Antonio (UTSA). I would also like to recognize the US Department of Education Undergraduate International Studies and Foreign Language Program Grant, which enabled me to carve out some time to direct my attention to this book when I was extremely busy directing the Medical Humanities Program at UTSA. I must also acknowledge my home institution, the Center for Bioethics and Humanities at the Norton College of Medicine at the State University of New York, Upstate Medical University, for giving me the space, freedom, and the Cbhonks support crew to focus on the book as I pushed over the finish line.

I have had the good fortune to be in constant contact with a bright, enthusiastic, and supportive international and interdisciplinary community of philosophers, psychiatrists, clinicians, and students, spanning my native Turkey and my found homes in Canada and the US. I am especially thankful to colleagues and friends who have been willing to read and discuss substantial parts of the project, especially Ken Schaffner, Clare Batty, Kathryn

Tabb, Jon Tsou, Peter Zachar, Robyn Bluhm, Jennifer Radden, Edouard Machery, Heather Douglas, Ginger Hoffman, Alicia Swan, M.J. Pugh, Bianca Zuniga, Sarah Robins, Corey Maley, Rachel Fabi, Liz Bowen, Syd Johnson, Meghan Page, Allison Krile Thornton, Collin Rice, and Kareem Khalifa who were the best interlocutors and cheerleaders as I wrote the book.

Earlier versions of the arguments presented in the book have benefited considerably from discussions at various conferences, including the meetings of the Association for the Advancement of Philosophy and Psychiatry, the Philosophy of Science Association, the Southern Society for Philosophy and Psychology, the American Psychiatric Association, and the American Philosophical Association. I am also grateful for the comments and feedback from the audiences in the invited talks I have given over the last few years at the University of Pittsburgh, the University of Waterloo, Purdue University, Michigan State University, the University of North Carolina Chapel Hill, the University of Cincinnati, and Tulane University.

I also owe my thanks and formal acknowledgment to several publishers for granting me permission to revise and republish parts of my own previously published work as follows:

Chapter 2 incorporates material from my 2014 article "Self-Insight in the Time of Mood Disorders: After the Diagnosis, Beyond the Treatment," published in *Philosophy, Psychiatry, and Psychology* 21(2), 139–155. All rights reserved.

Chapter 3 uses revised material in which I examine Ian Hacking's work from my 2016 article "Are Mental Disorders Natural Kinds?: A Plea for a New Approach to Intervention in Psychiatry," published in *Philosophy, Psychiatry, and Psychology* 23(2), 147–163. All rights reserved.

Chapter 6 is based on the arguments I have developed in my 2022 article, "Participatory Interactive Objectivity in Psychiatry," published in *Philosophy of Science* 89(5), 1166–1175. All rights reserved.

Chapter 7 uses material from a co-authored book chapter published in 2022 with Alicia Swan, Willie Hale, and M.J. Pugh. The chapter "Understanding Substance Use Disorders Among Veterans: Virtues of the Multitudinous Self Model," was published in *Evaluating the Brain Disease Model of Addiction*, edited by Nick Heather, Matt Field, Antony Moss, and Sally Satel, and published by Routledge Press, pp. 475–483. The data for the study that my colleagues and I conducted was collected thanks to the generous support by the Department of Veterans Affairs Health Services Research & Development Service (grant no. DHI 09–237) and the United Services Automobile Association, who provided the gift card incentive to survey participants. All rights reserved.

The biggest thanks go to my life partner, Jake Smith, for his constant patience, support, and enthusiasm for everything I do. He is the ocean to my rivers, the Adirondacks to my peaks. He is my anchor, my home.

Introduction

Mental distresses and disorders affect the individual as a whole and are expressed in the form of anomalies in self-related capacities and attitudes, such as self-control, self-conceptualization, self-respect, self-esteem, and self-efficacy. Not surprisingly, they often lead to the deterioration of individuals' relationships with themselves and others. For example, a woman diagnosed with post-traumatic stress disorder in the aftermath of a sexual assault while on the way home after an evening out with friends may blame herself for her choices (going out at night), in lieu of regarding the assailant as the single bearer of responsibility and blame. She may withdraw from socializing, especially at night. In fact, most mental disorders are expressed through turmoil in one's sense of self and ability to connect to others. They generate fractures in personal identity, i.e., characteristics that make a person who they are, and disruptions in the self, i.e., a dynamic, complex, relational, and multi-faceted system of mechanisms for capacities, processes, states, and traits supporting agency and autonomy.

Unfortunately, contemporary scientific psychiatry primarily engages with "mental disorders," not human selves. Most psychiatrists treat diseases, not people. A sophisticated and nuanced engagement with the self is missing from the standard scientific approaches to psychopathology. This undermines the importance of the self in both clinical and personal contexts, as the standard scientific frameworks not only guide clinical practice but also provide a medical and cultural framework to think about mental disorders. Although scientific and clinical discussions about psychopathology have forged links with philosophy of science and ethics, they have rarely benefited from a substantive engagement with cognitive sciences and empirically informed philosophical approaches to the self. *Reclaiming the Self in Psychiatry: Centering Personal Narratives for a Humanist Science* undertakes this project. Drawing on research in philosophy, psychiatry, cognitive sciences, medical humanities, and bioethics, I marshal their respective conceptual resources and develop a model of the self, the Multitudinous Self Model (*MuSe*), with the aim of facilitating the development of research to meet the clinical and conceptual needs of those touched by

DOI: 10.4324/9781003055556-1

mental distresses and disorders. The book humanizes psychiatry by putting the "self" at the center of contemplating mental disorders, while simultaneously redefining psychiatry's relationship with science as a care discipline.

Reclaiming the Self in Psychiatry: Centering Personal Narratives for a Humanist Science presents the problems created by the underappreciation of the self in contemporary scientific psychiatry and proposes solutions. More precisely, it identifies the need to make the self central to pragmatic approaches to mental disorders by means of a model of the self and proposes such a model. *MuSe* displays the complexity of the self and integrates three bodies of information to serve the clinical goals of psychiatry and provide conceptual and empirical tools for individuals responding to experiences of mental distresses and disorders. The three bodies are: 1) first-person reports or testimonies of those diagnosed with psychopathology that display the encounter with mental disorders; 2) empirical research on the self from the cognitive and behavioral sciences, such as psychology, sociology, and anthropology, reflecting the significance of biological, cognitive, social, and cultural factors shaping individuals' mental disorders; and 3) philosophical approaches to the self proposed by empirically informed philosophers.

My motivation to develop *MuSe* as a resource for the philosophical, scientific, clinical, and personal engagement with mental disorders came from years of experience, first, as a researcher whose gut instinct as a novice PhD student was to turn to first-person accounts to examine how mental disorders affect people and what it takes for diagnosed individuals to flourish; second, as a teacher in various institutions where I taught philosophy of science, medicine, cognitive science, and bioethics and mentored STEM students, medical humanities students, medical students, clinical psychology interns, and psychiatry residents; and third, as an empirically informed philosopher of mind and science trying to situate psychiatry among the sciences of the mind. In effect, I was simultaneously situated in three seemingly disparate worlds: one including patients whose direct encounter with mental disorders and the mental health system is overwhelming at best, and whose search for recognition and help is often unmet; one populated by well-meaning and enthusiastic students and professionals who genuinely want to help those experiencing mental distress and disorder by following a career in medicine; and one amidst philosophers of mind and science committed to understanding how cognition works *in situ*, and pursuing a more practice-oriented way of thinking about scientific activity by engaging with how science is practiced and how it relates and should relate to the public. I regularly wished for more communication, integration, and cross-fertilization between worlds, so that tools could be developed to guide well-meaning clinicians, the individuals themselves, and the scientific frameworks committed to enhancing psychiatry as a practice-oriented science. Developing a model of the self, *MuSe*, is my response. *MuSe* is designed to be an interface, a bridge, a connection between the more systematized and scientific strands of psychiatry exemplified by the classificatory framework of the Diagnostic and Statistical Manual of Mental Disorders (DSM), the art, skill, and know-how of the clinicians who treat patients, and the experience-based expertise of patients who encounter mental disorders and have much to say about what helps or impedes their flourishing.

There is a *prima facie* tension between psychiatry's commitment to adhering to the fundamental principles of science, such as validity, reliability, and generality, and paying closer attention to and taking seriously the patient or self-centered details of the encounter with mental disorders. In other words, the goal of pursuing objectivity seemingly precludes engaging with subjectivity. Contemporary scientific approaches in psychiatry have been looking for valid, reliable, and generalizable properties of mental disorders, avoiding self-related features and the particular contexts of those with a diagnosis because these efforts are seen as rejecting a scientific and objective framework. In *Reclaiming the Self in Psychiatry: Centering Personal Narratives for a Humanist Science*, I tackle this tension head-on and develop a framework for examining and treating mental disorders that is simultaneously self-centered and scientific. In other words, *MuSe* is intended to serve as a conceptual and empirical framework, not just for individuals to make sense of their mental distresses and disorders, not just for developing better clinical tools for their treatment, but also for housing, integrating, and making usable psychiatry's research findings. I emphasize the framework is not intended to rival other frameworks. The goal is simply to build bridges between various scientific and clinical approaches.

The book has two parts. In Part I, "The Missing Self in Psychiatry," I establish that the sophisticated complexity of the self is underexplored as a way to understand mental disorders in contemporary scientific psychiatry. To illustrate this, I focus on the DSM, the primary mental disorder classification system used in North America and around the world for scientific, clinical, administrative, and policy-related purposes. I zero in on the DSM's descriptions of three mental disorders: major depressive disorder (depression), substance use disorder (SUD), and post-traumatic stress disorder (PTSD). I highlight that these representations in the DSM focus on easily measurable and generalizable features and sidestep the complex and at times messy self-related phenomena that are indispensable for making sense of them. I invite the reader to approximate the first-person experience of these disorders by drawing on the memoirs of individuals with these conditions.

In this discussion, I access a wide range of mental disorder memoirs representing individuals with diverse backgrounds and experiences with mental health systems. I trace the historical evolution of the contemporary scientific framework, emphasizing psychiatry's twin commitments: first, to establishing itself as a legitimate scientific discipline, and second, to developing effective interventions into mental disorders that enable patients to flourish. I argue psychiatry's scientific aspirations to arrive at valid, reliable, and generalizable features of mental disorders and maintain scientific objectivity have inadvertently resulted in epistemic and ethical costs. I juxtapose the first-person accounts of mental disorders to the DSM's standardized descriptions to illustrate the DSM's frameworks are crucially incomplete. On the one hand, such incompleteness is expected and entirely natural when a system of representation tries to make a complex subject matter—mental disorders—scientifically tractable. On the other hand, ignoring the sophisticated complexity of selfhood when examining mental disorders runs the risk of not bringing clinically important information about mental disorders, via the self, to scientific, clinical, ethical, and personal realms. It is scientifically and clinically problematic, because the lack of a sophisticated engagement with the self draws an incomplete picture of mental disorders. It is epistemically and ethically costly from the perspective of the patient, as the DSM guides clinical practice, administrative decisions, policy, and the reflective frameworks in which individuals make sense of their condition. I propose rethinking and adjusting the scientific aspirations that have guided the development and use of the DSM, as well as revising its overreach, to better serve multiple goals of research, diagnosis, treatment, education, and policy.

In Part II, "Reclaiming the Self in Psychiatry," I develop *MuSe* to help psychiatry re-envision its scientific and clinical commitments. The fundamental intervention I offer here is that engaging with the self as a central framework for examining mental disorders does not violate psychiatry's scientific commitment to objectivity; in fact, it enhances it. Using insights from contemporary philosophy of science, I take psychiatry as a model-building science, according to which models enable access to complex real-world phenomena by highlighting certain specific aspects and making them amenable to manipulation. Embodying this vision, *MuSe* is designed to model the person, the subject of mental disorders. It can be used to display and organize the complexity of the self, making it a tool suitable for use by researchers, clinicians, and individuals with a mental disorder.

MuSe situates the self in the physical, social, and cultural environment and explores its complexity through five lenses: the *physical, experiential, social, conceptual,* and *narrative* attributes of the self. The model reflects the complexity of the self, including its dynamic interaction with the physical, social, and cultural environment and the capacities it supports, such as autonomy and agency. I remain agnostic on the nature of the self or its metaphysical structure. This book is not about what the self is, but rather how the concept of the self can be instrumentalized in the context of mental disorders. Thus, I use the concept of the self pragmatically.

MuSe is a model of the person and accounts for the experiences of "real people" as we encounter them in daily life, including those with and without psychopathology (Wilkes 1988). It draws on philosophy, social and cognitive sciences, and first-person reports to provide a framework for systematizing the dynamic complexity of the self and its relationships with physical, social, and cultural environments. The end goal is to integrate the seemingly disparate information about what it means to be a self, a person, to have a personal identity (using these concepts more or less interchangeably, noting their family resemblance) and use it when diagnosing, treating, researching, and reflecting on mental distresses and disorders.

Overall, *MuSe* provides empirical and conceptual resources that enhance how mental disorders are understood and treated by emphasizing the importance of and creating a pathway for integrating the first-person accounts of individuals with a mental disorder into knowledge-building practices in psychiatry. It does so by conceptualizing what it means to have a mental disorder and showing how the information from first-person testimonies can be organized and integrated. In this way, *MuSe* avoids the problems generated by mainstream psychiatry that are covered in Part I of the book. In addition, the model enhances psychiatry's twin commitments to scientific objectivity and patient flourishing, first, by showing how psychiatry can improve its relationship to science by adopting more expansive and sophisticated notions of expertise and objectivity, and second, by providing conceptual and empirical tools for clinicians and patients to respond to mental distresses and disorders. Notably, engaging with important work in feminist philosophy of science and epistemology, I propose some patients are experience-based experts whose contributions to reflections on mental disorders are indispensable, and I develop a conceptual framework for what I call participatory interactive objectivity in psychiatry.

I illustrate how the self-based framework can be applied to mental distresses and disorders by turning to SUDs. I show *MuSe* can provide clinical and reflective resources that will allow individuals with SUD to flourish. I bolster my arguments about the usefulness of the model for those with SUD by bringing together first-person narratives and relevant scientific and clinical work in psychiatry, cognitive sciences, and public health to shed light on some of the key scientific, clinical, and policy-related questions in psychiatry. My hope is that my application will invite other researchers to make use of and develop *MuSe* to address other mental disorders, such as attention deficit and hyperactivity disorder, PTSD, and depression. I conclude Part II with brief recommendations for philosophers, scientists, clinicians, clinical trainees, educators, patients, and policymakers, suggesting how the model can be developed and applied in conjunction with or separately from the existing frameworks in psychiatry.

Before closing, I must address the elephant in the room. The concept of the self has a bad reputation in philosophy because it is justifiably ambiguous and carries a lot of metaphysical baggage. A quick review of the history of philosophy reveals a host of self-deniers, self-skeptics, self-nihilists, and self-minimalists. Similarly, contemporary scientific psychiatry steers clear of the self because of what I dub the *Freud problem* in Chapter 2, i.e., an over-association of concepts like the self or person with psychoanalysis and a connected reluctance to engage with the self in the context of psychiatry because psychoanalysis is believed to be unscientific.

I disagree with this type of thinking. While it is beyond the scope of the book to engage with the important debate in philosophy on the metaphysics of the self, I will say this: The concept of the self is important, useful, and central to the ways we understand ourselves and connect to the world. The concept has been around since we were given the Delphic injunction to know ourselves and will always be there, regardless of metaphysical conundrums or post-Freudian scientific worries. In addition, a lot has happened since Freud, as I discuss in Chapter 4, and a person doesn't need to be a card-carrying psychoanalyst to work on and with the concept of the self. Notably, the cognitive revolution in the study of the mind and its processes rescued the research on human cognition from the grips of psychoanalysts and behaviorists in the 1950s. The self and various self-related concepts have been rigorously researched by cognitive and social scientists, informing empirically oriented philosophy of mind. Moreover, pragmatically speaking, the topic of the self is likely to remain one of the most popular subjects in philosophy, sociology, and psychology for students, teenagers, young adults, and people in various life stages and experiencing all types of crises. And popular culture's obsession with self-help—at least in Western, educated, industrialized, rich, and developed (WEIRD) (Henrich 2020) countries—is highly unlikely to disappear. Thus, leaning into the centrality and popularity of the concept of the self in folk psychology and popular culture, I highlight its scientific and clinical utility through the development of *MuSe*. Models in science are used to represent complex phenomena, without a particular commitment to those phenomena being "real" in a metaphysical sense. Similarly, I argue it is plausible to make use of *MuSe* in the context of psychiatry without any commitment to sorting out its reality or metaphysical structure.

My approach takes cues from Daniel Dennett's "intentional stance," i.e., his term for the level of abstraction involved in making predictions about the behavior of an intelligent agent by focusing on the agent's mental properties such as belief and desires. In an instrumentalist move, Dennett proposes it is best to understand complex systems, whether chess-playing computers or human agents, at the level of the intentional stance, without making a specific commitment to any deeper reality or metaphysical make-up of these systems (Dennett 1971). Dennett compares the intentional stance to physical and design stances. The physical stance makes predictions based on knowledge of the physical properties of the system and the natural laws that govern its operation, while the design stance makes predictions based on knowledge of things such as the purpose, function, and design of a system. Dennett argues the best chess-playing computers or human agents are practically inaccessible to prediction from either a physical or a design stance. Taking an intentional stance and considering mental states such as beliefs and desires will yield the most reliable predictions about human behavior.

In a similar move, I argue the concept of the self can be used to handle a lot of practical issues surrounding mental distresses and disorders. We do not need to settle on the metaphysical make-up of the self for the concept to be used in this way. For example, the concept of the self can be used to enrich one's conceptual framework in thinking about one's life experiences. Take the issue of personal reclamation; a self, say an individual with opioid use disorder, can reinvent and rebuild themselves by changing their self-narratives and self-concepts with the right kind of intervention. Thus, my concerns are scientific, clinical, medical, cultural, practical, and personal; in all these ways, the concept of the self is resourceful for responding to mental disorders.

To put it differently, my approach to the self and mental disorder embodies an approach to philosophy of science that directly engages with practice and practical problems. Often called philosophy of science in practice, this approach highlights the need for philosophers to study scientific practices to advance their understanding of the relationship between scientific theories and the world (Hacking 1983; Ankeny et al. 2011). This means philosophers of science should acknowledge scientific practices are shaped by scientific practitioners and the social and cultural circumstances in which they are situated, and the development of scientific knowledge is intimately tied to these practices (Potochnik 2017). Philosophy of science in practice calls for the inclusion of practicing scientists and policymakers in philosophical conversations about the nature and applications of science, while encouraging "them to become more reflective about their practices, as well as the underlying assumptions and the implications of these practices" (Ankeny et al. 2011). Heeding the call, I aim to build a bridge between philosophy of science and practitioners in mental healthcare by focusing on practices of knowledge development and use in psychiatry and considering the impact of these practices on individuals diagnosed with mental disorders. I am interested in bringing the practical aspects of not quite fitting in, of living with a mental disorder, of its diagnosis and clinical treatment, to the attention of practitioners in mental healthcare, so that they become more reflective about their underlying assumptions about mental disorders and see the impact of their knowledge-building practices on those diagnosed with a mental disorder. I look at practices of knowledge-building in psychiatry through a detailed investigation of the DSM's practices, supplementing this with an examination of the first-person reports of those diagnosed with mental disorders. A focus on psychiatry's knowledge-building practices makes explicit the various assumptions, intentions, and oversights of the field, and a focus on testimonies shows how these affect individuals' responses to their mental disorders. In addition, testimonies demonstrate how resourceful and important it is to give uptake to the voices of those with experience-based expertise and position them on the same platform as other experts.

As I develop in Chapter 5, a distinction between mental distress and mental disorder is important, and a mental disorder diagnosis does not necessarily and consistently help the individual with mental distress. This is why a close analysis of an individual's encounter with psychiatric practice is necessary. *MuSe* is grounded in the rich tradition of selfhood found in philosophy, science, and the humanities. As such, it provides a language with which to think about mental distress or disorder, ultimately enhancing individuals' agency and autonomy and supporting their flourishing. While I do not engage with the rich philosophical literature on flourishing for reasons of scope and space, in what follows, I define flourishing as the development of an individual's psychological and social skills to facilitate relationships with the self and others in the face of the challenges inherent in physical, social, and cultural environments. Deciding what counts as flourishing for an individual is a matter of negotiation that includes the individual in question. However, as I point out in the Epilogue, putting the self at the center of engaging with mental distresses and disorders will enable psychiatry to benefit from the philosophical literature on concepts such as agency, autonomy, and flourishing as it develops more effective interventions into mental disorders.

In conclusion, the self is not an idle concept philosophically, scientifically, clinically, or ethically; it does important regulatory and normative work in organizing human experience and proliferating moral possibilities. If we know the characteristics of the self, we may be able to improve the lives of those whose self-experiences are not conducive to flourishing. The conceptual and practical resourcefulness of *MuSe* will help medical students and psychiatry residents better connect their medical and scientific training to their clinical encounter with patients; it will give clinicians tools to navigate the self-related disruptions in their patients; it will give researchers measurable targets to understand the cognitive, social, and cultural factors that shape psychopathology; it will empower individuals diagnosed with mental disorders to respond to the states of affairs pertaining to their disorders in the broader context of their selfhood and their visions of flourishing; finally, it will support communication between philosophers of psychiatry, researchers who work on sciences of the mind, patients with direct encounter of mental disorders, and scientists and clinicians who are sensitive to the first-person encounters of mental disorders. Simply stated, *MuSe* offers resources for psychiatry to reinvent itself as a simultaneously scientific *and* humanistic discipline. The model can help psychiatry update and expand its understanding of what it means to be scientific by redefining its central concepts such as expertise and objectivity, while also recognizing that in so far as it is a care discipline that aims to help people with mental disorders live better lives, it needs to do a better job of engaging with what it means to be a human, aligning itself with areas of inquiry such as medical humanities that situate health and illness in the life of a person, society, environment, language, and culture.

References

Ankeny, Rachel, Hasok Chang, MarcelBoumans, and Mieke Boon. 2011. Introduction: Philosophy of Science in Practice. *European Journal for Philosophy of Science* 1 (303). doi:10.1007/s13194-011-0036-4.

Dennett, Daniel C. 1971. Intentional Systems. *Journal of Philosophy* 68, 87–106. doi:10.2307/2025382.

Hacking, Ian. 1983. *Representing and Intervening: Introductory Topics in the Philosophy of Natural Science*. Cambridge: Cambridge University Press.

Henrich, Joseph. 2020. *The WEIRDest People in the World: How the West Became Psychologically Peculiar and Particularly Prosperous*. New York: Farrar, Straus, and Giroux.

Potochnik, Angela. 2017. *Idealization and the Aims of Science*. Chicago: University of Chicago Press.

Wilkes, Kathleen. 1988. *Real People*. Oxford: Oxford University Press.

Part I

Chapter 1

Mental disorder and the self

1.1 Introduction

This chapter provides a snapshot of what it is like to have a mental distress or mental disorder in the words of patients themselves and shows what we miss if we do not engage with these self-stories. It draws attention to discrepancies between depictions of mental disorders in contemporary scientific frameworks and personal testimonies by analyzing the representations of mental disorders in the Diagnostic and Statistical Manual of Mental Disorders (DSM), widely used in the United States and around the world for various scientific, clinical, administrative, policy-related, and educational purposes, and the reports of first-person encounters with mental disorders in the memoirs of individuals diagnosed with a mental disorder. Section 2 provides an overview of how mental disorders are accounted for in scientific frameworks, such as the DSM, on the one hand, and in testimonial frameworks, such as the memoirs of individuals with mental struggles, on the other hand. Section 3 reviews the first-person testimonies of five patients with various mental struggles and mental disorders, with close attention to their words, and juxtaposes them to the ways their mental disorders are represented and characterized in the DSM. The chapter concludes by analyzing why the first-person accounts of mental disorders are indispensable for psychiatry's scientific and clinical goals and calls for building bridges between scientific and testimonial frameworks of mental disorders in contemporary mental healthcare. Such bridge-building is necessary to reinvent psychiatry as a simultaneously scientific and humanistic area of inquiry.

1.2 Two pictures of mental disorders

This chapter juxtaposes two pictures of mental disorders. One picture maps mental disorders using the language of the contemporary scientific approach in psychiatry, i.e., by listing mental disorder symptoms (observed and reported by patients) and signs (observed and reported by others) as these appear in the DSM, the dominant scientific framework that guides clinical,

DOI: 10.4324/9781003055556-3

administrative, policy-related, educational, and conceptual decisions about mental disorders, not just in the US but around the world. The second picture uses individuals' own words, their descriptions of "what it is like" for them to feel different and to have mental health struggles, to live with depression, substance use disorders, or trauma. These first-person testimonies demonstrate how mental disorders compromise the person as a whole, through the deterioration of self-related capacities and attitudes. Self-related phenomena, such as negative self-feelings, diminished sense of self-worth, destabilized self-concepts, and challenges to self-control, are all important instigators of or contributors to an individual's encounter with mental disorder. Clinicians must acknowledge and engage with these phenomena to develop effective interventions so patients can flourish, despite the constraints associated with mental disorders.

In juxtaposing the scientific framework to the testimonial framework, my goal is to illustrate that scientific frameworks such as the DSM unavoidably fall short of fathoming the complexity of first-person encounters with mental disorders, and contemporary psychiatry needs conceptual and practical tools to better engage with the self-related dimensions of the encounter with a mental disorder to help people get better and flourish. The DSM framework falls short because it focuses on patients' observable behavior, i.e., symptoms and signs—for the purposes of easing scientific discovery—and this undermines the experiential and conceptual thickness and complexity of the self that is the subject of the mental disorder. The DSM does not intend to sidestep the self, or at least, it does not have an explicit agenda to overlook the complexity of the persons it wants to treat. However, because it is a scientific framework, and scientific frameworks, in a bid to maintain objectivity, often seek to provide a bird's-eye view of the phenomenon under scrutiny, searching for regularities and arriving at generalizable features of that phenomenon, the DSM misses important self-related features of mental disorders that cannot be captured by the insular language of signs and symptoms.

As we will see in subsequent chapters, since its inception in the early 1950s, the DSM has been pursuing a scientific agenda, looking for mechanisms underlying and managing mental disorders—whether brain mechanisms, genetic lineage, or medications—with the goal of developing effective clinical interventions. This search has not always been fruitful for the individual who urgently needs help and does not have the luxury to wait until mechanisms are identified by science, if ever. More importantly, because the DSM-oriented scientific inquiry has primarily looked for large-scale regularities and interventions, it has lost sight of the particular yet empirically tractable details about individuals: what makes them who they are, how their cognition works, how they journey through time, how they develop and maintain social relationships, how their bodies and physical environments change, and how mental disorders intersect not only with the flesh of their being but also with the social and cultural environments in which they are embedded.

In contrast, first-person testimonies of mental health struggles take us deep inside the subject, or the person, or the self who is touched by a mental disorder. We join these subjects to see what happens to them: how they feel and think about the experience, how the experience is entrenched within their social relationships, cultural backgrounds, and fears and excitement about the future, and how they respond, including how they create a niche and learn to flourish despite their mental disorder. Patients' self-related capacities and attitudes, as well as other self-related contingencies, such as their race, gender, socioeconomic status, and personal identity—i.e., what makes us who we are and distinguishes us from others—are important in understanding both the onset and the course of a mental disorder and developing resources useful to the clinicians who treat these patients. It is crucial, for example, for the clinician to understand how a person who was subject to sexual assault assigns self-blame for what happened, thus exacerbating their post-traumatic stress disorder (PTSD), if that clinician is to provide help.

Beyond their utility to the clinician, self-based frameworks and tools are crucial for individuals to make sense of their mental disorder-related experiences and to develop psychological and social resources that will enable flourishing. In the context of this book, I define "flourishing" broadly, as the development of subjects' psychological and social skills in interpreting and judging their relationships with themselves and others in the face of the circumstances in which they are placed, the demands of the world, and the challenges they are subject to therein. The acquisition of psychological and social skills that promote "agency," i.e., individuals' capacity to act in the world as subjects, and "autonomy," i.e., their ability to make informed and uncoerced decisions related to the states of affairs in their life, is closely connected to their flourishing. These skills enable them to live a responsible and fulfilling life, in which they are accountable for their decisions and actions, follow through with their commitments to themselves and others, and take ownership of their mistakes.

What is revealed in first-person testimonies is not a part of the DSM-style scientific picture of mental disorders, and we need tools that build bridges between the two, if the goal of the science of mental disorders is to help individuals flourish. The DSM's (inadvertent) sidestepping of the self-related features of the encounter with mental disorder has been costly in epistemic, clinical, ethical, and personal contexts, largely because of the ubiquity of the DSM in the US and around the world, including for research, diagnosis, treatment, insurance, administrative, policy-related and educational purposes. The ways mental disorders are delineated in the DSM's scientific framework mean these concepts and frameworks play a crucial role in many contexts; they are used to guide clinicians' treatment decisions, to determine whether certain interventions are covered by insurance, to determine eligibility for leave time from work, to establish the kind of education students receive in medical schools and other healthcare professions training, and to dictate how patients understand and respond to their experiences with their mental disorder. The DSM's extended reach, as will be further examined in the following chapter, combined with its perhaps expected or legitimate limitations as a scientific representational system, has had epistemic, clinical, ethical, and personal costs.

The good news is that there are ways for the DSM or other scientific frameworks to engage with self-related properties of mental disorders to develop effective and ethical clinical interventions that will help patients flourish. This book tells that story. *Reclaiming the Self in Scientific Psychiatry: Centering Personal Narratives for a Humanist Science* tracks the epistemic, clinical, ethical, and personal costs of ignoring the self-related properties of mental disorders and offers a strategy to enhance psychiatric epistemology, aid clinical encounters, and help persons with mental distress flourish. I invite psychiatry, as an area of inquiry into mental disorders, to engage with the full complexity of the self by turning to people's own stories and also to the sciences that study people (e.g., psychology, sociology, anthropology, cognitive science, etc.), to develop tools to help people in distress. To aid psychiatry in pursuing this goal, in Chapter 4, I develop the Multitudinous Self Model (*MuSe*) and demonstrate how it supports flourishing.

Before moving further, let's settle on the terminology. Going against the traditional philosophical trend, throughout the book, I use interchangeably the concepts of the self, personal identity, person, and subject (of mental disorder). Since the Delphic injunction to "know thyself," the concept of the self has played a prominent role, not just in philosophy, but also in other mind sciences such as psychology, anthropology, sociology, and cognitive sciences at large. Philosophical debates center on metaphysical questions about whether the self is real, epistemological questions about how it can be known, and practical and ethical questions about self-directed feelings and attitudes, such as self-respect. In the cognitive sciences, most of the focus has been on self-related and empirically tractable phenomena, including self-related feelings such as self-confidence, self-esteem, and self-efficacy. There is a similarly large philosophical literature on concepts such as personhood and personal identity. Philosophers debate what it means to be a person, whether the body is needed for the characterization of personhood (e.g., Locke), whether chimpanzees are persons (e.g., Andrews et al. 2018). There are also questions about what it means to have a personal identity, whether it is best characterized in the re-identification sense—asking under which conditions a subject at one point in time can properly be re-identified at another point in time—or in the characterization sense, asking under which conditions various experiences, psychological characteristics, and actions are properly attributable to a particular person (Schechtman 1996). The answers to these questions have practical bearings on moral questions, such as responsibility and blame. When we turn to other sciences, such as sociology, personal identity plays an important role in characterizing an individual's situatedness in a social and cultural world on the basis of intersectional characteristics, such as gender, sexuality, race, socioeconomic status and education levels.

Ultimately, I perceive this group of concepts to have a family resemblance in the Wittgensteinian sense, especially when making sense of mental disorders (Wittgenstein 1953). All these concepts—the self, person, subject, and personal identity—are connected by a series of overlapping similarities, and they are all affected or compromised by the encounter with a mental disorder. Simply put, the self or the person is the subject of the mental disorder, and the mental disorder experience is intimately tied to an individual's personal identity, say, as a teenager or an immigrant. And when individuals with a mental disorder commit a crime, they have to face the law with the recognition that they may or may not have the full capacity to stand trial.

Thus, my reasons to use these concepts interchangeably, in their chaotic and messy forms, are pragmatic. I am not interested in thought experiments about persons to nail down a philosophical nuance. Rather, I want to examine what happens to "real people" (Wilkes 1988) when they are touched by a mental disorder. What happens to real people when they have mental distress or disorder is always entrenched in their past, their personal history, their self-related feelings and attitudes, the kinds of persons they are perceived to be in a particular society and culture, and their freedom and responsibility. While there are robust reasons to draw distinctions between these concepts in the philosophical terrain of getting a grip on "people," for the purposes of this book, these distinctions are limiting. The world of real people is not very neat or organized, but it is rich and important, and all these concepts help draw the complex picture of mental disorders. In fact, not centralizing the linguistic, experiential, and conceptual complexity of these self-related concepts to make sense of mental disorders has been costly, not just for the science of psychiatry but also for the development of clinical interventions that aid patients to recover and flourish.

Let's look at the costs of side-stepping the complexity of selfhood when making sense of mental disorders. Some of these will be apparent later in the chapter in the stories of individuals whose lives are touched by mental disorders, as they tell us in their own words about the struggle to make sense of their experiences, participate in daily life, and find ways to flourish, either withstanding or recovering from their mental disorders. Epistemic costs are mostly knowledge-related. Because the self-related features of the encounter with mental disorders are not part of the scientific framework, attempts to know more about them through scientific research have yielded limited results. For example, once highly touted pharmacological approaches to mental disorders, which focus on targeting the brain mechanisms associated with mental disorders to provide treatment, in lieu of focusing on the self as a whole, do not seem to be meeting the needs of individuals. Notably, major pharmaceutical companies are deemphasizing or exiting psychiatry (Hyman 2012). This is because, in the words of Steve Hyman, the former director of the National Institute of Mental Health (NIMH), compared to other fields of medicine, psychiatry has found "few, if any, validated molecular targets, and this makes it hard to define criteria for molecular target validation for human brain disorders" (Hyman 2012). He adds that the animal-based assays used in new drug development have failed to identify efficacious drugs with new molecular mechanisms, "and given scant understanding of the pathophysiology of common psychiatric disorders, it is difficult to develop better models" (Hyman 2012). Epistemic costs have ripple effects in the clinic because scientific frameworks shape clinical interventions; if the self-related features of mental disorders are not thoroughly examined in the scientific context, it is challenging for clinicians to come up with interventions that directly target the patient's concerns in the clinic, and it is challenging for patients to negotiate a treatment plan that will guide them as they navigate their mental health struggles. Clinicians are increasingly recognizing that psychotropic medications alone are limited in their effectiveness: they do not help all patients, and to the extent that they do, they have multiple undesirable side effects.

Epistemic and clinical costs have ethical consequences: clinicians cannot meet their ethical responsibility to do the most good for the person who is suffering, because they do not have the clinical tools to engage with self-related aspects of an individual's encounter with mental disorders. Patients, in turn, might feel they are not being heard, because clinicians think their self-related struggles have no place in clinical encounters. In addition, the DSM-style conceptual framework that is disseminated through the institutional structures governing mental healthcare (from hospitals to medical schools, healthcare professional programs, media, and beyond) shapes the ways individuals make sense of their mental disorders. On the one hand, they may get the help they need; on the other hand, they may overidentify with their diagnosis in ways that impede their flourishing (Tekin 2011). In this way, the DSM-style scientific frameworks can be personally costly for those who want to flourish. To summarize, these costs are failure to make progress in identifying the causes of mental disorders, failure to identify effective treatments, failure to help patients understand and manage their experience of disorders.

How can we build bridges between the DSM-style scientific framework of mental disorders and the persons the framework intends to help? My solution involves engaging robustly with the self that is the subject of mental disorders. This chapter outlines the first step towards making the self central in psychiatry: turning to the subjects themselves and listening to their testimonies. The first-person testimonies[1] of mental struggles provide unique resources for psychiatry and are indispensable to attempts to find tools to help individuals flourish. In the following section, I give examples to make my case, including testimonies about major depressive disorder (depression), substance use disorder, and PTSD. Some of these first-person accounts come from a time when different scientific frameworks were dominant, while others reflect the contemporary state of affairs in psychiatry. They all point to the thickness, messiness, and density of the first-person encounter with mental disorder. They all illustrate the costs of not embracing the complexity of the self.

1.3 What is it like?

1.3.1 Misdiagnosis

Janet Frame, the world-renowned author from New Zealand, was hospitalized in a psychiatry unit as a young girl for what she describes as "being different" (1982, 229). Frame's autobiography, *An Angel at My Table,* is packed with vivid descriptions of her childhood and her family's hardships: her family was poor, her brother had epilepsy, her two sisters both drowned, and she was different:

> To be different was to be peculiar, a little "mad."... [W]hen I was asked about my reading and I ... mentioned a novel few had heard of, the teacher would again say "Jean's so original." Therefore, in an adolescent homelessness of self, in a time where I did not quite know my direction, I entered eagerly a nest of difference which others found for me but which I lined with my own furnishings; for, after all, during the past two years I had tried many aspects of "being"—a giggling schoolgirl who made everyone laugh with comic recitations, mimicry, puzzles, mathematical tricks, ... and now I was at home, with some prestige and fairly comfortable.
>
> (Frame 1982, 113)

Frame's response to being different and labelled as such was to embrace and customize her difference and create a little world for herself in the nook of difference. She talks about her loneliness at a teachers' training college and says she found peace sitting in a cemetery among tombstones. Around this time, when she was doing her teaching practicum as a part of her teacher training, she panicked when an inspector entered the classroom to observe her teaching. She fled the classroom and never returned. Soon after, she attempted suicide and spent the following eight years in mental hospitals in New Zealand, receiving electroshock treatments over two hundred times. She was about to have a lobotomy, the operation where the nerve fibers in the prefrontal area of the brain are cut, once regarded as a groundbreaking psychiatric treatment, but she was released from the hospital when a hospital official discovered she had won a literary prize. Her writing literally helped her regain her freedom and autonomy.

Frame tells the story as follows. Her mother was "persuaded" to sign a permission for her to undergo leucotomy/lobotomy (Frame 1982, 229). The decision for the operation came after what Frame calls the experts' "heavily wielded arguments" in support of the operation (1982, 230). Speaking of these experts, Frame says:

> [They were] the experts who over the years as my "history" was accumulating, had not spoken to me at one time for longer than ten or 15 minutes, and in total time over eight years, for about 80 minutes; who had administered no tests, not even physical tests of EEG or X-rays; the experts whose judgment was based on daily reports by overworked irritable nursing sisters. I listened, … when Dr. Burt, a likeable overworked young doctor who had scarcely spoken to me except to say "good morning, how are you" and not wait for a reply as he was whisked through the ward, found time to explain that I would be having a leucotomy operation, that it would be good for me, that, following it, I would be "out of hospital in no time." I listened also with a feeling that my erasure was being completed when the ward sister, suddenly interested that something was about to be "done" with and to me, painted her picture of how I would be when it was "all over." "We had one patient who was here for years until she had a leucotomy. And now she's selling hats in a hat shop. I saw her just the other day, selling hats, as normal as anyone. Wouldn't you like to be normal?" Everyone felt that it was better for me to be "normal" and not have fancy intellectual notions about being a writer, that it was better for me to be out of hospital, working at an ordinary occupation, mixing with others.
> (Frame 1982, 230)

As the narrative makes clear, Frame's agency and autonomy were undermined in the clinical context, and the complexity of who she was, what her life story was like, what exactly her problems were, and what led her to run away from the classroom and attempt suicide were never really engaged with in the clinic. Agency refers broadly to the manifestation of the capacity to act and make decisions regarding one's life. She was not treated as an agent, an expert on her own life or mental states, as evident by the fact that no one in the clinic bothered to ask what was wrong with her or consulted her on what she wanted or needed. At the same time, she was not able to exercise her autonomy, i.e., use her agency to make decisions about her treatment. It was assumed she could not make such decisions (undermined agency), and the clinicians knew what was good for her (undermined autonomy).

Against this clinical backdrop, Frame was scheduled for a lobotomy. One evening, the hospital superintendent walked into Frame's room; she was expecting him to talk about the operation, but that was not the case. Pointing to a newspaper in his hand, he told Frame that her book *The*

Lagoon had won the Hubert Church Award for the best prose and was mentioned in the *Star* newspaper. He had therefore decided to move her out of the ward and cancel the lobotomy. As Frame puts it, her "writing saved" her:

> I repeat that writing saved me. I had seen in the ward office the list of those "down for leucotomy," with my name on the list, and other names being crossed off as the operation was performed. My "turn" must have been very close when one evening the superintendent of the hospital, Dr. Blake Palmer, made an unusual visit to the ward. He spoke to me—to the amazement of everyone. As it was my first chance to discuss with anyone, apart from those who had persuaded me, the prospect of my operation, I said, urgently, "Dr. Blake Palmer, what do you think?" He pointed to the newspaper in his hand. "About the prize?" I was bewildered. What prize? "No," I said, "about the leucotomy." He looked stern, "I've decided that you should stay as you are. I don't want you changed." He unfolded his newspaper. ... "You've won the Hubert Church Award for the best prose. Your book, *The Lagoon*." ... I smiled. "Have I?" "Yes. And we are moving you out of this ward. And no leucotomy."
>
> (Frame 1982, 230–231)

She was later discharged from the hospital and carried on with her life as an aspiring young writer. Frame's story warns mental health professionals to avoid a false diagnosis that could lead to erroneous and even harmful medical treatment. She was (mis)diagnosed with a mental disorder, owing partly to clinicians' failure to understand the reasons for her suicide attempt and to recognize her dream of becoming a writer as a worthwhile ambition. Her difference from others, set against an underprivileged background, led others to assume she was mentally ill. Frame's story also gestures to the tight connection between various aspects of her personhood, including her passion for writing, her creation of a world for herself through words, her sense of difference, loneliness, and isolation, and her time in a psychiatric hospital. Her story tells the tale of a socially and psychologically struggling young woman from a poor family, who, once she finds her niche, flourishes and becomes a well-known writer who connects with and inspires others. When she won a prize for her writing, others realized that her experience— her madness, if you will—was not without reason. There was something unique about her, and she did something well. She wrote an award-winning book; thus, there were reasons for clinicians to keep her as she was and allow her to stay unchanged.

Frame's story is illustrative of the complexity of the self, the person who is the subject of mental struggles, and it shows how failing to engage with its complexity might lead to misdiagnosing idiosyncratic states of being as mental disorder and prescribing medical interventions that are impossible to undo. More importantly, the story emphasizes how strengthening individuals' agency and autonomy will help them cope with the challenges in their lives, whether mental disorders or other kinds of challenges, paving the way for their flourishing.

1.3.2 Diagnosis as death sentence

Elyn Saks is a successful professor of law, diagnosed with schizophrenia. She was first treated by a medical professional when she was an undergraduate at Oxford. At this time, she received psychoanalytic treatment. Her condition was later diagnosed as schizophrenia, under the DSM classification. When Saks read the description of schizophrenia in the DSM, she was startled:

> I had discovered the DSM. ... I read it cover to cover. Knowledge had always been my salvation, but with my immersion into the DSM, I began to understand that there were some truths that were too difficult and frightening to know. ... And now, here it was, in writing: The Diagnosis. What did it mean? Schizophrenia is a brain disease which entails a profound loss of connection to reality. It is often accompanied with delusions, which are fixed yet false beliefs—such as you have killed thousands of people—and hallucinations, which are false sensory perceptions—such as you have just seen a man with a knife. Often speech and reason can become disorganized to the point of incoherence. The prognosis: I would largely lose the capacity to take care of myself. I wasn't expected to have a career, or even a job that might bring in a pay check. I wouldn't be able to form attachments, or keep friendships, or find someone to love me, or have a family of my own—in short, I'd never have a life. ... I'd always been optimistic that when and if the mystery of me was solved, it could be fixed; now I was being told that whatever had gone wrong inside my head was permanent, and from all indications, unfixable. Repeatedly, I ran up against words like "debilitating," "baffling," "chronic," "catastrophic," "devastating," and "loss." For the rest of my life. The rest of my life. It felt more like a death sentence than a medical diagnosis.
>
> (Saks 2007, 167–168)

Note that the description of schizophrenia in the current edition of the DSM (DSM-5) does not contain all these phrases and descriptions, and it is unclear which edition Saks read. But we should minimally trust that something Saks read in the DSM and/or cognate sources led her to frame the diagnostic nomenclature in those terms. For example, while this way of thinking about schizophrenia is not a part of the diagnostic criteria for schizophrenia in the DSM-5, the schizophrenia section contains statistical information on the kinds of impairments people might experience. The section on the "Functional Consequences of Schizophrenia" says the following:

Schizophrenia is associated with significant social and occupational dysfunction. Making educational progress and maintaining employment are frequently impaired by avolition or other disorder manifestations, even when the cognitive skills are sufficient for the tasks at hand. Most individuals are employed at a lower level than their parents, and most, particularly men, do not marry or have limited social contacts outside of their family.

(American Psychiatric Association 2013, 104)

There is a good chance that Saks synthesized the DSM information with accounts of schizophrenia that are popular in the media (e.g., schizophrenia as a brain disorder) to arrive at her interpretation of schizophrenia as a death sentence. A diagnosis that was intended to help her get access to what she needed to get better was not helpful to her. Instead, she had to find her own ways of making sense of what was happening to her and develop strategies to flourish as a person. Her memoir explains how she achieved this: she obtained meaningful work, cultivated strong relationships, found clinicians who engaged with her, and created a niche for herself.

Saks' story illustrates two things. The first is that the DSM description is incomplete, and as it is a simplified version of a complex phenomenon, it is susceptible to being misinterpreted and miscommunicated. It is true that some individuals who have schizophrenia feel debilitated and have difficulty maintaining relationships or holding jobs. However, it is not necessarily the essential characteristic of the condition that would hold for everyone under every circumstance—and the DSM does not say that it does. In fact, empirical evidence suggests with the right kind of support and by strengthening their agency, people with the most severe mental disorders can create a meaningful life, including work and personal relationships (Harrison et al. 2001; Rosen 2006; Tekin and Outram 2018). Yet it seems the limitations and imperfections of diagnostic descriptions were not communicated to Saks, and this negatively affected her self-concept and the way she thought about herself. She came to think of her mental disorder as a death sentence; she thought she would "largely lose the capacity to take care of" herself and was not "expected to have a career, or even a job that might bring in a pay." She had hallucinations, as outlined in the DSM, but determining whether these were "catastrophic" or "debilitating" required her to have a conversation with her clinician on what this experience meant to her and the ways to think and not think about the DSM framework. But this did not happen.

The problem here is not the DSM's description of schizophrenia but how its incompleteness is communicated to and received by the patient. In an ideal world, whatever the DSM says would have been delivered in a careful and nuanced way, and Saks would have been given the tools to understand her diagnosis and contextualize it in the larger complexity of her life, negotiating and developing the ability to deal with her hallucinations so that the diagnosis would lead to flourishing, not to a death sentence.

Consider another example of the limitations of the DSM framework. One of the symptoms of schizophrenia listed in the DSM is "affective flattening, alogia, or avolition," defined as lacking interest in social relationships (American Psychiatric Association 2013). However, persons with schizophrenia report that it is not really about a lack of interest in social relationships; rather, they point to an intense desire but perceived inability to initiate and build such relationships (Parnas and Henriksen 2014). As this example suggests, the DSM's disorder descriptions are not fully representative of an individual's lived experiences.

What ultimately helped Saks to flourish and to meet the challenges of her experience with schizophrenia was not the prescriptive and narrow narrative of a DSM diagnosis but her ability to find a line of work that satisfied her and to develop meaningful social connections and a personal support system. Saks writes at length about how studying philosophy and having a job she loves help her function and cope with her schizophrenia: "Everyone has a niche. Of course, resources are heavily skewed against the mentally ill, and the majority never have a chance to realize anywhere near their potential" (2007, 334). Saks acknowledges that an individual's work environment may need to be adapted to a lower level of functioning and states explicitly that not every individual diagnosed with schizophrenia or another mental disorder can become successful in their career, but everyone should be able to find something they enjoy and earn a livelihood (Saks 2007).

Some might argue that patients simply misinterpret these diagnostic descriptions, and the DSM is not intended to be used by the patients themselves in this manner. I will engage with this topic in the following chapters, but for now, it is sufficient to say that unfortunately, as clearly stated in the introductions to the DSM-III, DSM-IV, and the DSM-5, the manual is designed to guide not only diagnosis and treatment but also scientific, administrative, policy-related and educational practices involving mental disorders. Moreover, the DSM shapes both the public understanding of what mental disorders are and individuals' understanding of their own mental disorders. Given the self-reflective nature of human cognition and the ways social and cultural environments influence our narratives about ourselves, thinking about our experiences through the language of the DSM is neither implausible nor wrong; it is just the human propensity to make sense of things. We need tools to build bridges between scientific and testimonial frameworks so that the former are responsive to individuals' need to flourish.

1.3.3 Color of depression

In her memoir, *Willow Weep for Me: A Black Women's Journey Through Depression* (1998), Meri Nana-Ama Danquah, a Ghanaian-American writer, describes the complex relationship between her encounter with depression and her identity as a Black immigrant woman who survived domestic abuse.

She writes that the financial and emotional responsibilities as a single mother taking care of her child and as a writer with an unsteady income played a role in the onset of her depression and shaped her response to it— for better or worse. She contextualizes this observation in relation to her personal history. She moved to the US from Ghana when she was six to live with her mother, who had immigrated three years earlier to attend Howard University. Danquah's loneliness and isolation as an immigrant Black girl in the US were exacerbated by her parents' divorce. Stresses did not end when she became an adult. While she was happy to become a mother, her partner was abusive, and she had to file a restraining order against him because of domestic violence. At the same time, she was trying to build a career as a writer and coping with clinical depression.

Danquah's encounter with depression cannot be untangled from her self-hood or personal identity, i.e., what makes her who she is. This means the constituents of her personal identity in the characterization sense (Schechtman 1996), including her race, gender, socioeconomic status, and social relationships, played a role in the onset and development of her depression. For example, she writes about the challenges of being an immigrant, caught between two cultures. She was often torn, she says, between the "rigid mores" of the Ghanaian culture and "the overly permissive attitudes of Americans" (Danquah 1998, 33–34). Conflicts between these cultural norms had a direct impact on her self-concept, especially in a school with no other Black students. She was always considered a "foreigner," and she "hated being different":

> I used to come home from school and stand in front of the mirror and practice talking like the kids in school. Walking like them. Hell, I wanted to be them. All I knew was that I had to be someone other than who I was.
>
> (Danquah 1998, 91)

When the emotional work of trying to fit in was combined with the stress of her parents' divorce, the situation worsened:

> Long after my father moved out, I used to sit by that window in the evenings, waiting for his car to roll into the lot, waiting for him to come back home. When night had finished falling and he hadn't returned, the despair cut so deeply, I thought it would slice me in half. This is the first clear memory I have of feeling overwhelmingly sad for a lengthy period of time, of hating myself so much that I wanted to die.
>
> (Danquah 1998, 106)

This is the experience of a young child who feels lost, lonely, and isolated at home because of her parents' divorce and who feels different from other children because she is a Black immigrant girl. The narrative highlights Danquah's feelings of abandonment and loneliness, as she grappled with her father's absence. She seems to have responded to this traumatic event by blaming herself for the divorce. Her relationship with herself in these formative years was shaped under these circumstances, and she started developing destructive self-criticism. On top of all these internal conflicts and tensions, she was raped by her mother's boyfriend when she was a teenager, and this led to a suicide attempt. Trying to adjudicate the tensions and conflicts between herself and the world strained her mental health; she started developing an extreme "self-hate" (Danquah 1998, 91).

Danquah's choices and actions as an adult, the relationships she formed, and most importantly for present purposes, her mental health problems are best understood in relation to her unique history and experiences. Consider gender. She writes that hormonal changes during and after pregnancy exacerbated her depressed mood, eventually leading to what was diagnosed as post-partum depression. Next, consider her relationships: she found herself in an abusive relationship and encountered domestic violence but ultimately left her partner. Life remained full of challenges, however, as she was a single mother. Her productivity as a writer declined, she doubted her writing skills, and she struggled financially. Consequently, her sense of self-efficacy, i.e. her belief in her capacity to meet the demands of the world (Bandura 1977), shrank.

This example shows how factors constituting Danquah's identity led to a decline in her mental health. Carrying the sole responsibility of parenting, ranging from the daily tasks of childcare, such as preparing breakfast and taking the child to school, to the emotional responsibilities involved in raising a child, impoverished her emotional resources and likely contributed to the development of depression. She found herself attracting "unhealthy relationships" and inadvertently subjected herself and her already "battered" self-image to additional abuse: "It is like a self-fulfilling prophecy" (Danquah 1998, 41). The more she became subject to abuse by others, the more she engaged in self-abuse.

Paradoxically, these dimensions of her self-experience, from her physical realities to her relationships and self-concepts, also enabled her "to move past the temptation" to go "right back into bed" (Danquah 1998, 17). They helped her develop resilience and respond more effectively to her depression. She says being a mother affected the way she related to herself and how she took care of herself. Even in the darkest times of her depression, even when she wanted to run away from her responsibilities, she was fully aware that she could not abandon her daughter, nor could she "drape her body in thick blankets, toss her over her shoulder" like some "runaway's sack" and take her with her (Danquah 1998, 16). Her daughter's reliance on her and her ability to cope helped Danquah hold on to her life despite the darkness she was feeling.

Racial identity also played an important role in Danquah's encounter with depression. She talks about the challenges of being a Black woman in mostly white communities. In addition, she suggests the norms in the Black community about mental health problems hindered her ability to ask for help. Danquah says she had to hide her depression from her community and avoided seeking help for a long time because she was afraid of being misunderstood, losing friends, and losing the respect of her community. One reason for her "prolonged silence" about her depression was what she perceived to be the Black community's expectations of Black women:

> The illusion of strength has been and continues to be of major significance to me as a black woman. The one myth that I have had to endure my entire life is that of my supposed birthright to strength. Black women are supposed to be strong—caretakers, nurturers, healers of other people—any of the 12 dozen variations of Mammy. Emotional hardship is supposed to be built into the structure of our lives. It went along with the territory of being both black and female in a society that completely undervalues the lives of black people and regards all women as second-class citizens. It seemed that suffering, for a black woman, was part of the package.
>
> (Danquah 1998, 19)

The conflict between Danquah's self-concept as a person struggling with mental health issues and her perception of her community's expectations of Black women as strong, resilient, and tough exacerbated her depression and prevented her from reaching out for help, at least initially. When she did talk to others, her experiences were not positive:

> I have had conversations about my depression with black people—both men and women ... I've frequently been told things like: "Girl, you've been hanging out with too many white folk"; "What do you have to be depressed about? If our people could make it through slavery, we can make it through anything"; "Take your troubles to Jesus, not to damn psychiatrist."
>
> (Danquah 1998, 20)

Thus, the combination of stereotypes about mental illness and stereotypes about the strength of Black women influenced her encounter with depression and her ability to seek help or develop effective responses. Danquah says:

> Stereotypes and cliches about mental illness are as pervasive as those about race. I have noticed that the mental illness that affects white men is often characterized, if not glamorized, as a sign of genius, a burden of cerebral superiority, artistic eccentricity—as if their depression is

somehow heroic. White women who suffer from mental illness are depicted as idle, spoiled, or just plain hysterical. Black men are demonized and pathologized. Black women with psychological problems are certainly not seen as geniuses; we are generally not labeled "hysterical" or "eccentric" or even "pathological." When a black woman suffers from a mental disorder, the overwhelming opinion is that she is weak. And weakness in black women is intolerable.

(Danquah 1998, 20)

She dives deeper into this point when she compares her depression to that experienced by William Styron, a fiction writer and essayist. She points out that her experience is significantly different from the depression of Styron, simply because he is a privileged white male:

Like Styron and I would never have the same angle on anything. We had the same illness; the similarities end there. The way I did depression was a whole 'nother bag of beans. I'm a single black mother about a half paycheck away from the government cheese line.

(Danquah 1998, 235)

Her personal situation influenced the way she conceptualized and responded to her depression, including her difficulty finding a conceptual and communal space within which to reflect on her unique experience with depression. She had difficulty, for example, defining what her depression felt like in a way that did justice to her experience:

You've heard descriptions of depression before: A black hole; an enveloping darkness; a dismal existence through which no light shines; the black dog; darkness; and more darkness. But what does darkness mean to me, a [Black] woman who had spent her life surrounded by it? The darkness of my skin; the darkness of my friends and family. I have never been afraid of the dark. It poses no harm to me. *What is the color of my depression?*

(Danquah 1998, 22; emphasis added)

It is important to recognize that Danquah's experience of depression and her response to it were molded not just by the unique aspects of her personal identity but also by her physical, social, and cultural environment. All of these dimensions of her encounter yield important information about the fabric of Danquah's experience. Understanding this tapestry is essential in the clinical context to help her respond to her circumstances and allow her to flourish.

What is also noteworthy is that Danquah experienced tensions and conflicts between different self experiences. Socially, she was trying to fit into the Black community, but she was not happy about the community's perception of her depression and wanted to distance herself so that she could get the help she needed, further complicating her experience of depression. Danquah conceptualized these conflicts and contradictions when she started writing about her depression: a process she calls the "writing cure" (1998, 128). Weaving together the conflictual yet consistent threads of her encounter with depression in a particular niche helped her embrace her personal journey and opened a space in her own conceptual and experiential world.

Now, let's return to the project of juxtaposing this thick self-narrative of depression to the way depression is characterized in the DSM. According to the DSM-5, the diagnostic criteria for major depressive disorder are the following: five or more of the identified symptoms have been present during the same two-week period and represent a change from previous function, and at least one of the symptoms is either "(1) depressed mood or (2) loss of interest or pleasure" (DSM-5 2013, 160). Other symptoms include significant weight changes, sleep problems, psychomotor agitation and retardation that is "observable by others, not merely subjective feelings of restlessness or being slowed down," fatigue, feelings of worthlessness or guilt, diminished ability to think or concentrate either by subjective account or as observed by others, and recurrent thoughts of death or a suicide attempt (DSM-5 2013, 160–161). In addition, these symptoms must cause clinically significant distress and impairment in social and occupational areas of functioning, and they are not explained by schizoaffective disorder.[2]

There is a significant difference between the description of depression in the DSM manual and Danquah's first-person account. Danquah's story is thick, packed with details, contexts, people, and geographies. She tells us a causal story, specifying what led to what. She contextualizes, for instance, her inability to get out of bed, saying what eventually helped her was her love for her daughter. She explains in detail how her culture made her reluctant to seek help. The DSM language is thin, clean, straightforward, and unbothered by messy details. The reason is simple: the DSM is a diagnostic and clinical guide and a scientific tool, as stated clearly in its introduction. It aims to be used as a research and clinical tool, with applications in educational and policy-making contexts. It purports to provide objective criteria for mental disorders and thus refers to behaviors using objective parameters, such as observability by self and others, and generalizability to the experience and behavior of a population of individuals, not just one. For example, if a person experiences insomnia every day, this can be verified by people sharing a house with them. This description results in a more generic account of depression. "Of course," we might say, "that's the goal." It is generic so that it can be used to understand a large group of individuals with similar experiences.

My worry is that when the DSM is used as a tool by the clinician to diagnose and treat the individual's condition, its lack of detail creates impediments to the full understanding of the individual's personal encounter and precludes effective treatment. It gives little guidance on how to look for the specific features and experiences of the person, even though understanding these is necessary for treatment. The clinician needs the details of insomnia or the contexts for feelings of guilt or reluctance to seek help if they want to guide recovery. In addition, DSM-style descriptions of mental disorders influence the way individuals understand their condition and how they respond to it. There must be a bridge between the testimonial and scientific frameworks.

1.3.4 Substance use and denial

Now we turn to Caroline Knapp's story of her life as a "high-functioning alcoholic" (Knapp, 1996). In *Drinking: A Love Story* (1996), Knapp examines her alcohol use, saying her "love affair" with alcohol threatened to destroy her own life and the lives of others. Her excessive drinking almost caused the death of a friend's two young daughters (Knapp 1996, xv), and she holds herself fully responsible. She focuses on what it was like to live with alcohol use disorder,[3] providing a detailed account of her intense cravings, her denial of the problem, and the strategies she used to drink in a socially acceptable manner without raising alarm bells. For example, at work, she would wait impatiently for happy hour so she could drink under the guise of socializing. She always had a few more drinks than others. She drank a bit more as she drove home (she kept a bottle in her car) and continued to drink at home. She characterizes her "descent" into alcohol use disorder as a loss of control (Knapp 1996).

Knapp's substance use was intimately tied to her personal identity and social relationships. She outlines how her family life and romantic relationships contributed to her drinking. Her father tended to make her feel exposed and anxious, so instead of asking for and receiving love from him or her other loved ones, she drank to feel happier and more relaxed so that she could be more likable. Drawing an analogy between alcohol cravings and hunger, she explains she had a strong, persistent neediness she just couldn't ignore, just like when she was hungry:

> Alcoholism feels like the culmination of ... dozens of tiny fears and hungers and rages, dozens of experiences and memories that collect in the bottom of your soul, coalescing over many many many drinks into a single liquid solution.
>
> (Knapp 1996, 74)

One of the interesting insights we get from Knapp's story is her account of denial: denial that she has a drinking problem, denial that she needs help, denial that her substance use hinders her flourishing. Denial is one of the most pervasive features of substance use disorders and one of the leading reasons people do not seek help, or do not follow through with a plan of treatment when they do seek help. For example, for a long time, Knapp rationalized her (excessive) alcohol use by finding someone with a more severe drinking problem to compare herself to. For years, this helped her think that her drinking was not a cause for alarm.

Knapp says there is usually a long decline before reaching the bottom. For Knapp, this began with her father's death. Watching her father's illness shut down one part of his body after another was devastating for her. At the end, she reports, his memory and personality disappeared. Her father's death was followed by her mother's illness, accompanied by anxiety-provoking tests and nightmarish hospital visits. This made Knapp's alcohol use disorder worse:

> During both illnesses, and after both deaths, I drank with the no-holds-barred abandon of the truly self-pitying drinker, every night until I passed out ... [but] what stands out are a few key scenes, ones that had less to do with the facts of illness and loss than with what I was forced to see through those experiences about myself.
>
> (Knapp 1996, 219)

We also discover in Knapp's memoir what eventually helped her quit drinking: joining an Alcoholics Anonymous (AA) group and receiving therapy. AA groups are part of an international organization founded in 1935 to provide emotional and practical support for people with substance use disorders. They encourage participants to follow a spiritually inclined 12-step program to help them abstain from substance use and maintain sobriety. Knapp's account of her experience in rehab and her early trips to AA meetings shows how she regained control of her life by learning to tolerate difficult emotions and to address problems rather than waiting for someone else to do it. In the final chapter of her memoir, she reflects on the perspective she gained by becoming sober, especially by interacting with a supportive community of AA attendees.

Knapp's story of her struggle with and recovery from addiction is detailed and thick, packed with details of the factors that contributed to her addiction: her upbringing, her emotional development, the family's ways of giving and receiving love, and so on. It also gives a sense of what it was like for her: the denial, the planning, the cravings, the ways alcohol made her feel safer or more fun, her self-reflection as she descended to the bottom—where she finally found the strength to "move up!"

These details are important. They are important for the scientist who is doing research on the role of denial in addiction or is interested in the full spectrum of the stages of craving. They are also important for clinicians or family members—they will better understand the stages of denial and thus be better able to help. Finally, the details are important for self-reflective, reason-responsive agents who want to understand and respond to their own struggle with substance use.

Now let's see how the DSM describes alcohol use disorder. First, it specifies there must be a pattern of alcohol use occurring within a year that has led to clinically significant impairment, manifested by at least two of the following symptoms: behavioral patterns, such as alcohol being taken in larger amounts or over a longer period than was intended; persistent desire or unsuccessful efforts to cut down or control consumption; significant time spent in activities necessary to obtain and use alcohol or recover from its effects; recurrent alcohol use resulting in a failure to fulfill major obligations at work, school, or home. In addition, clauses in the diagnostic criteria indicate the harms of alcohol use: continued use of alcohol despite social or interpersonal problems caused or exacerbated by its effects; reduction in social, occupational, or recreational activities as a result of alcohol use; and continued use despite knowledge of a persistent or recurrent physical or psychological problem likely to have been caused or exacerbated by alcohol. Finally, the DSM specifies biological markers for diagnosis, such as increased tolerance and withdrawal symptoms.

It is noteworthy that the DSM's description of alcohol use disorder provides indicators and risk factors that go beyond behavioral and biological markers to include race, gender, and ethnicity. For example, it lists prevalence rates among racial and ethnic subgroups of the US population. For 12- to 17-year-olds, rates are higher among Hispanics (6 percent) and Native Americans and Alaska Natives (5.7 percent), and lower among whites (5 percent), African-Americans (1.8 percent), and Asian-Americans and Pacific Islanders (1.6 percent). For adults, the 12-month prevalence of alcohol use disorder is greater among Native Americans and Alaska Natives (12 percent) than among whites (8.9 percent), Hispanics (7.9 percent), African-Americans (6.9 percent), or Asian-Americans and Pacific Islanders (4.5 percent). The DSM-5 also lists risk factors for alcohol use disorder, including genetic, physiological, and environmental aspects. However, it still lacks the kind of contextualized details required to understand the experience of alcohol use disorder, the kind we encounter in Knapp's memoir. The DSM offers a clear picture that may be helpful for diagnosis, but not for the full clinical treatment—nor will it help an individual with the disorder to find useful tools. Once again, we need a bridge between the scientific and testimonial frameworks.

1.3.5 Trauma and the self

Susan Brison, a philosophy professor, has written about her experience of post-traumatic stress disorder (PTSD), a mental health condition caused by an extremely stressful event that an individual has witnessed or directly experienced. In 1990 Brison was sexually assaulted in France during a morning walk. Her attacker severely beat her and strangled her to unconsciousness, leaving her to die. The experience "destroyed" her world, she writes (Brison 1996, 2002). She subsequently used her training as a philosopher to tell the story of what this experience did to her sense of self and personal identity and how she flourished in its aftermath. Brison reflects on the experience of trauma by citing Judith Herman, who says a traumatic event "destroys the belief that one can be oneself in relation to others" (quoted in Brison 2002, 14). To this, Brison adds that one can no longer maintain one's relationship with oneself, since this relationship is intimately tied to one's relationship with others.

Brison says the assault affected her as a whole, including her self-narratives and her autonomy, writing that the "pleasures of embodiment were replaced by the pain and terror to which being embodied makes one prey" (1992, 16). Just prior to the assault, Brison was contemplating pregnancy and thinking about her body in the process of becoming a mother. All those feelings were replaced by the feeling that her body was just a "prey" (Brison 1992, 16). She emphasizes that memories are physiological trauma; they linger in the body long after the event, recurring "either as full sensory replay of traumatic events in dreams or flashbacks, with all things seen, heard, smelled, and felt intact or as disconnected fragments" (Brison 1992, 17).

For a long time after the attack, Brison was not able to go for a walk alone because she was afraid. She also cut her hair so that she did not look like a woman from behind. Similar experiences have been reported by other victims of trauma, she notes, such as Holocaust survivors:

> The human ritual of renewal meant relearning old habits from her "former" or pre-Auschwitz life: how to use a toothbrush, toilet paper, handkerchief, knife, and fork; how to smile, first with the lips, then with the lips and eyes; how to recapture forgotten odors and tastes, like the smell of rain. Implicit in the procedure of renewal, however, annealed to it with the epoxy of disruptive memory, is the "counter-time" of Auschwitz, where the rain stank of diarrhea and beat down on the camp, the victims, "the soot of the crematoriums and the odor of burning flesh."
>
> (Langer 1991, 3)

Another dimension of the embodied experience of trauma that Brison high-lights, connecting it to her own experience, is bodily dissociation. Adults who are sexually assaulted sometimes "split" from their bodies, or at least separate from their former selves after the attack. Some cope by giving themselves new names. This is observed among Holocaust victims as well. One writes:

> No doubt, I am very fortunate in not recognizing myself in the self that was in Auschwitz. To return from there was so improbable that it seems to me I was never there at all. ... I live within a twofold being. The Auschwitz double doesn't bother me, doesn't interfere with my life. As though it weren't I at all. Without this split I would not have been able to revive.
>
> (Delbo 1985, 2; quoted in Brison 1992, 19–20)

Brison highlights the intrinsic social dimensions of her experience with trauma and recovery. She writes that during an attack, victims confront a social death as much as a physical one and can only be "resurrected ... with the help of others." Brison mentions the first-person account of Jean Améry, the Austrian-born writer tortured by the Gestapo, who makes a similar point about his trauma: "From the moment of the first blow,'" he says, the victim loses "trust in the world," including "the irrational and logically unjustifiable belief in absolute causality perhaps, or the likewise blind belief in the validity of inductive inference" (Améry 2009). According to Améry, victims experience the loss of certainty that others will continue to respect their physical and metaphysical being.

Brison describes how the experience of sexual assault and the following trauma interrupted her self-narrative by breaking the continuity in her memories, almost leading to the creation of a self distinct from her former selves. The event disrupted her vision of the future because her traumatic memories (especially perceptual and emotional flashbacks) felt "passively endured;" she lacked control and conscious choice—both of which are pre-requisites for a narrative. Yet Brison says it is possible to learn to control one's own narrative of trauma; in fact, that is how one restores one's sense of self. At the same time, though, the narrator requires a listener: Brison's recovery was possible with the help of others, even though the trauma was caused by others. She defines what she calls the "Necessity of the Empathic Other," whereby "in order to recover from trauma, the survivor needs to construct a narrative and tell it to an empathic listener, in order to re-externalize the event" (Brison 1992, 26).

Brison also describes the effect trauma had on her autonomy, her capacity to make decisions for herself. Trauma undermined her autonomy because she experienced the feeling of having lost control of her environment and what happened to her body. She considers this a radical transformation, in that the pre-trauma self is almost a completely different person from the post-trauma self. Thus, she defines the recovery process, or at least her recovery process, as having three components: regaining control of the self, regaining control of the environment, and reconnecting with humanity. Whether the latter two happen, Brison writes, is contingent on the survivor's social environment—on other people. Finally, Brison says having a child helped her regain her autonomy. Citing Jennifer Nedelsky, Brison writes that the experience of childbearing encapsulated "the emergence of autonomy through relationship with others" (Brison 2002).

Now, let's turn to how PTSD is described in the DSM-5. According to the DSM, there are five categories of experience that must be individuated through five criteria, each of which includes a cluster of symptoms. Criterion A is exposure to death, serious injury, or sexual violence by: 1) directly experiencing the traumatic event(s); 2) witnessing, in person, the event(s) as it occurred to others; 3) learning from a violent or accidental traumatic event(s) as it occurred to someone close; or 4) experiencing repeated or extreme exposure to aversive details of the traumatic event(s) (e.g., first responders collecting human remains; police officers repeatedly exposed to details of child abuse). Criterion B is the presence of one (or more) intrusion symptoms associated with the traumatic event(s), beginning after the traumatic event(s) occurred, including: 1) recurrent, involuntary, and intrusive memories about the event; 2) recurrent distressing dreams in which the content and/or affect of the dream is related to the traumatic event(s); 3) dissociative reactions (e.g., flashbacks) in which the individual feels or acts as if the traumatic event(s) were recurring; 4) intense psychological distress at exposure to internal or external cues that symbolize an aspect of the traumatic event(s); or 5) marked physiological reactions to internal or external cues that symbolize or resemble an aspect of the traumatic event(s). Criterion C is the persistent avoidance of stimuli associated with the traumatic event(s), beginning after the traumatic event(s) occurred, as evidenced by one or both of 1) avoidance of or efforts to avoid distressing memories, thoughts, or feelings about or closely associated with the traumatic event(s); and 2) avoidance of or efforts to avoid external reminders (people, places, conversations, activities, objects, situations) that arouse distressing memories, thoughts, or feelings about or closely associated with the traumatic events. Criterion D refers to the existence of negative alterations in cognitions and mood associated with the traumatic event(s), beginning or worsening after the traumatic event(s) occurred, expressed as: 1) the inability to remember an important aspect of the traumatic event(s); 2) persistent and exaggerated negative beliefs or expectations about oneself, others, or the world (e.g., "I am bad;" "No one can be trusted;" "The world is completely dangerous;" "My whole nervous system is permanently ruined"); 3) persistent, disordered cognitions about the cause or consequences of the traumatic event(s) that lead individuals to blame themselves or others; 4) persistent negative emotional state (e.g., fear, horror, anger, guilt, or shame); 5) markedly diminished interest or participation in significant activities; 6) feelings of detachment or estrangement from others; 7) persistent inability to experience positive emotions (e.g., happiness, satisfaction, or loving feelings). Criterion E is the presence of marked alterations in arousal and reactivity, evidenced by two or more of the following symptoms: irritable behavior and angry outbursts, reckless or self-destructive behavior, hypervigilance, exaggerated startle response, problems with concentration, or sleep disturbance. The disturbances listed in Criteria B–E must be present for a month, must cause clinically significant distress or impairment in social, occupational, or other areas of functioning, and must not be attributable to the physiological effects of a substance (e.g., medication, alcohol) or another medical condition. In some cases, PTSD symptoms might be co-present with dissociative symptoms, such as depersonalization (American Psychiatric Association 2013, 271–272).

The list of PTSD diagnostic criteria in the DSM-5 is comprehensive and includes different ways individuals encounter its symptoms. Yet the descriptions are dry, and they lack detail, especially when contrasted to Brison's account. When we read Brison's account, we get a robust sense of the way trauma is entrenched in all aspects of Brison's being, and we also learn what may help people like her. In contrast, the DSM gives a broad characterization of PTSD, but falls short of provide tailored roadmap that can be used to guide the patient. Once again, we need a bridge between the scientific framework and the testimonial framework to benefit the clinical context.

1.4 Conclusion

This chapter has juxtaposed scientific and testimonial frameworks of mental disorders to highlight the ability of first-person testimonies to enhance the understanding of mental disorders in a way that improves interventions and enables flourishing. A close reading of five memoirs has revealed the richness of an individual's experience with mental disorder, highlighting its entrenchment with various self- and identity-related features of the individual's life. The analysis has also illustrated how individuals' perceptions of their encounter with a mental disorder help them find the tools they need to flourish, despite their condition. The analysis leads to three conclusions.

First, the experience of (putative) mental disorder is complex, largely because it is tightly woven into the experience of the self as whole, in its full complexity. The encounter with a mental disorder and its related phenomena is not easily separable from the self; there are intrinsic ambiguities between self-experience and disorder experience—also dubbed self-illness ambiguity (Dings 2020; Dings and De Bruin 2023; Dings and Glas 2020; Jeppsson 2022; Sadler 2007; Tekin 2022). The illness experience is shaped by the self-experience, and the self-experience is shaped by the illness experience. A thorough understanding of mental disorders requires the engagement of the complexity of the self or personhood or personal identity. This is important for the ways individuals make sense of their experiences and, as such, can assist clinicians who are trying to help them improve their mental health and functioning. Unless the mental disorder experience is tied to the fabric of the self of the patient, effective and ethical treatments are unlikely to be found, and patients' flourishing can be blocked.

Second, first-person testimonies provide a wealth of information that could and should guide clinicians and patients in developing tools for flourishing. As mentioned earlier in the chapter, I define "flourishing" as the development of individuals' psychological and social skills in interpreting, judging, and reasoning out their relationships with themselves and others in the face of their present circumstances and challenges and the demands of the world. The acquisition of psychological and social skills that promote "agency," defined as the capacity to act in the world as a subject, and "autonomy," defined as the capacity to make informed and uncoerced decisions related to the states of affairs, are closely connected to flourishing. They enable the individual to establish a responsible and fulfilling life, despite mental disorder.

The six narratives covered in this chapter tell stories of flourishing. They involve individuals who are different and do not quite fit into their social environments. They have complex but not uncommon personal histories involving loss, immigration, poverty, violence, and lack of love. As the narrators search for mental healthcare and recovery, they have experiences of unbecoming, not being understood, supported, or aided. In the end, they all more or less learn to live with their mental struggles and even flourish. They are actively involved in rebuilding themselves, cultivating nurturing relationships, and shaping their physical, social, and cultural environments in a way that centralizes their personality, identity, and meaning. Their stories invoke the cognitive niche construction theory in cognitive science, according to which organisms are not just shaped by their physical, social, and cultural environments but also shape and transform these environments in ways that facilitate (or sometimes impede) their persistent individuation and survival. This theory recognizes the centrality of environmental resources to human intelligence and suggests many organisms intervene in their environment and shape it in ways that improve the adoptive fit between the agent and its world (Sterelny 2010). This construction of a cognitive niche simplifies the environment and allows the development of cognitive power in a way that enhances day-to-day problem-solving resources (Stotz 2010). The testimonies show how these individuals created and nurtured a niche and made possible the creation of a meaningful life.

Third, we have had a glimpse into how contemporary DSM-style scientific frameworks for mental disorders do not engage deeply with the richness of the self- or person-related aspects of mental disorders. For example, the DSM draws a map of mental disorders based on a simplified account of behavioral symptoms and signs and stays away from things like the context in which they emerge, how they mesh with the person as a whole, and so on. As we will see in Chapters 2 and 3, the DSM stays away from those details because it aims to provide observable and generalizable features of disorders applicable to a large population of individuals, not just one person. However, because there is no other context in which these person- or self-related details are reintroduced in clinical treatment plans, important self-related conceptual and empirical resources are underutilized. The DSM diagnostic criteria are not simply tools for organizing and categorizing human experience; they are also clinical and educational tools for developing successful treatment. However, successful treatment rests on a systematic engagement with the self-related complexities of mental disorders. We need to find a way to bring the self into discussions about treatment and flourishing.

Notes

1 I use "self-reports," "testimonies," and "first-person accounts" interchangeably.
2 The DSM-5 also identifies possible risk and prognostic factors, including temperament such as neuroticism or negative affectivity, as well as environmental factors, such as childhood experiences, and genetic and physiological course modifiers, etc.
3 Knapp refers to her experiences as "addiction," echoing the philosophical debates on addiction (Flanagan 2013a, 2013b; Pickard and Ahmed 2019; Tekin 2019; Tekin, Flanagan, and Graham 2017). However, instead of "addiction," I use "substance use disorder," for three reasons: 1) substance use disorder is associated with a list of diagnostic criteria in the DSM-5, and the DSM framework of mental disorders is a core focus in this book; 2) substance use disorder is linked to degrees of severity (mild, moderate, and severe in DSM-5), whereas addiction suggests a binary of addicted and non-addicted and overlooks the nuances between the two extremes; and 3) the label "addict" is highly stigmatizing but likely to be used when the term addiction is adopted. The second reason is important here, as I claim significantly reducing the severity of a disorder is a compelling reason to see a medical intervention as an effective treatment.

References

American Psychiatric Association. 2013. *Diagnostic and Statistical Manual of Mental Disorders (DSM-5)*. Washington, DC: American Psychiatric Publishing.

Améry, Jean. 2009. *At the Mind's Limits: Contemplations by a Survivor on Auschwitz and Its Realities*. Bloomington, IN: Indiana University Press.

Andrews, Kristin, Gary Comstock, G.K.D. Crozier, Sue Donaldson, Andrew Fenton, Tyler John, L. Syd, M. Johnson, Robert Jones, Will Kymlicka, Letitia Meynell, et al. 2018. *Chimpanzee Rights: The Philosophers' Brief*. London: Routledge.

Bandura, A. 1977. Self-Efficacy: Toward a Unifying Theory of Behavioral Change. *Psychological Review* 84(2), 191–215.

Brison, Susan. 1996. Outliving Oneself: Trauma, Memory and Personal Identity. In *Feminists Rethink the Self*, edited by Diana T. Meyers. Boulder, CO: Westview Press.

Brison, Susan. 2002. *Aftermath: Violence and the Remaking of a Self*. Princeton, NJ: Princeton University Press.

Danquah, Meri Nana-Ama. 1998. *Willow Weep for Me: A Black Women's Journey Through Depression*. New York: Norton.

Delbo, Charlotte. 1985. *Days and Memory*. Translated by Rosete Lamont. Marlboro: Marlboro Press.

Dings, Roy. 2020. *Not being Oneself? Self-ambiguity in the Context of Mental Disorder*. PhD dissertation. Radboud University Nijmegen.

Dings, Roy and L.C. De Bruin. 2023. Self-illness Ambiguity and Narrative Identity. *Philosophical Explorations* 26(2), 147–154.

Dings, Roy and Gerrit Glas. 2020. Self-Management in Psychiatry as Reducing Self-Illness Ambiguity. *Philosophy, Psychology & Psychiatry* 27(4), 333–347.

Flanagan, Owen. 2013b. "Identity and Addiction: What Alcoholic Memoirs Teach." In *The Oxford Handbook of Philosophy and Psychiatry*, edited by K.W.M. Fulford, M. Davies, R.

Flanagan, Owen. 2013b. The Shame of Addiction. *Frontiers in Psychiatry* 4, 120.

Frame, Janet. 1982. *An Angel at My Table*. New York: George Braziller, Inc.

Gipps, G.Graham, J.Z.Sadler, G.Stanghellini, and T. Thornton, pp. 865–888. Oxford: Oxford University Press. Harrison, G., K. Hopper, T. Craig, E. Laska, C. Siegel, J. Wanderling, K.C. Dube, K. Ganev, R. Giel, W. van der Heiden, S.K. Holmberg, A. Janca, P.W. Lee, C.A. León, S. Malhotra, A.J. Marsella, Y. Nakane, N. Sartorius, Y. Shen, C. Skoda, R. Thara, S.J. Tsirkin, V.K. Varma, D. Walsh, and D. Wiersma. 2001. Recovery from Psychotic Illness: A 15- and 25-year International Follow-up Study. *The British Journal of Psychiatry: The Journal of Mental Science* 178, 506–517.

Hyman, Steven E. 2012. Revolution Stalled. *Science Translational Medicine* 4(155), 1–5.

Jeppsson, Sophia. 2022. Solving the Self-illness Ambiguity: The Case for Construction over Discovery. *Philosophical Explorations* 25(3), 294–313.

Knapp, Caroline. 1996. *Drinking: A Love Story*. New York: Random House Publishing Group.

Langer, Lawrence. 1991. *Holocaust Testimonies: The Ruins of Memory*. New Haven, CT: Yale University Press.

Parnas, J. and M. G. Henriksen. 2014. Disordered Self in the Schizophrenia Spectrum: A Clinical and Research Perspective. *Harvard Review of Psychiatry* 22(5): 251–265.

Pickard, Hanna and Serge Ahmed. 2019. *The Routledge Handbook of Philosophy and Science of Addiction*. London: Routledge.

Rosen, Alan. 2006. Destigmatizing Day-to-Day Practices: What Developed Countries can Learn from Developing Countries. *World Psychiatry* 5(1), 21–24.

Sadler, John Z. 2007. The Psychiatric Significance of the Personal Self. *Psychiatry* 70 (2), 113–129.

Saks, Elyn R. 2007. *The Center Cannot Hold: My Journey Through Madness*. New York: Hachette Books.

Schechtman, Marya. 1996. *The Constitution of Selves*. Ithaca, NY: Cornell University Press.

Sterelny, Kim. 2010. Minds: Extended or Scaffolded?. *Phenomenology and the Cognitive Sciences* 9, 465–481.

Stotz, Karola. 2010. Human Nature and Cognitive–Developmental Niche Construction. *Phenomenology and the Cognitive Sciences* 9, 483–501.

Tekin, Şerife. 2011. Self-Concept through the Diagnostic Looking Glass: Narratives and Mental Disorder. *Philosophical Psychology* 24(3), 357–380.

Tekin, Şerife. 2021. Is Big Data the New Stethoscope? Perils of Digital Phenotyping to Address Mental Illness. *Philosophy and Technology* 34, 447–461.

Tekin, Şerife. 2022. My Illness, My Self, and I: When Self-narratives and Illness-Narratives Clash. *Philosophical Explorations* 25(3), 314–318.

Tekin, Şerife, Owen Flanagan, and George Graham. 2017. Against the Drug Cure Model: Addiction, Identity, and Pharmaceuticals. In *Philosophical Issues in Pharmaceutics: Development, Dispensing, and Use*, edited by Dien Ho, pp. 221–236. Dordrecht: SpringerNetherlands.

Tekin, Şerife and Simon Michael Outram. 2018. Overcoming Mental Disorder Stigma: A Short Analysis of Patient Memoirs. *Journal of Evaluation in Clinical Practice* 2(5), 1114–1119.

Wilkes, Kathleen V. 1988. *Real People: Personal Identity Without Thought Experiments*. Oxford: Clarendon Press.

Wittgenstein, Ludwig. 1953. *Philosophical Investigations* (3rd ed.). Translated by G. E.M. Anscombe. New York: Macmillan.

Chapter 2

Psychiatry and science

2.1 Introduction

Contemporary psychiatric research on mental disorders has twin commitments: one is clinical, and the other is scientific. First, as a branch of medicine, psychiatry has a pragmatic clinical commitment to alleviate the burden of mental disorders on individuals so affected. Mental disorders are problems for the individuals experiencing them, their loved ones, and the larger society, and as such, they call for the development of clinical interventions[1] that help these individuals flourish, by either full recovery or enabling them to live a life that is fulfilling despite the constraints of a mental disorder. Second, psychiatry has a commitment to scientific objectivity: interventions into mental disorders must be grounded on valid scientific constructs of mental disorders, and they must be reliable enough to be used as treatments for populations of individuals with mental disorders, as opposed to being sporadically helpful for a few individuals.

In this chapter, I show the contemporary framework for mental disorders falls short of simultaneously meeting the scientific and clinical goals of psychiatry. Psychiatry's attempts to establish itself as a legitimate scientific discipline that meets the ideal of objectivity have resulted, albeit inadvertently, in sidestepping the self as a target of inquiry, leading to a framework for care that is not fully responsive to the needs of patients. Section 2 provides a history of the evolution of the contemporary scientific framework, emphasizing its twin scientific commitments: to develop effective interventions into mental disorders that help patients flourish and to arrive at an objective framework to investigate mental disorders. Section 3 examines the features of the current scientific framework for mental disorders. Section 4 illustrates that contemporary psychiatry suffers from twin failures: the descriptions of mental disorders in terms of behaviors are isolated from the integrated complexity of the self who encounters them, leading to an incomplete picture, and the ability of self-reports to add to scientific research is underappreciated, resulting in missed opportunities to develop effective treatments. As further developed in Chapter 3, the twin failures have undermined the self in scientific and clinical contexts, with epistemic and ethical costs.

DOI: 10.4324/9781003055556-4

I use the Diagnostic and Statistical Manual of Mental Disorders (DSM) as the primary document to trace the evolution of psychiatry's twin commitments for strategic reasons. A historical analysis of this document by focusing on the revisions since its inception in 1952 (as I do in this chapter) helps track psychiatry's scientific aspirations and understand the sources of its scientific (and political) authority. In addition to serving as the primary document for the classification of mental disorders in the United States and around the world for scientific research, clinical diagnosis, clinical treatment, education, and various administrative and policy-related purposes, the DSM provides an important source of information about mental disorders to patients and the public at large, thus shaping the culture of mental health and disorders. Although it originated in the United States, the DSM is widely used in research and clinical contexts, including in Canada, Australia, Japan, Korea, Taiwan, and Turkey (Kuroki et al. 2016; Suzuki et al. 2010). Some critics even argue the DSM-style of thinking about mental disorders and mental health practices has been "globally exported," and this has obscured the importance of engaging with cultural variations and differences to understand mental disorder and mental health (Watters 2010).

Further, the DSM framework has been influential in the distribution of funding for research on mental disorders. For example, the National Institute of Mental Health (NIMH), as the provider of the largest amount of funding for research on mental disorders in the US and the world (with a budget of US$2.54 billion in 2024), determines which areas of research must be prioritized to understand and treat mental disorders, and until recently, it used the DSM criteria for mental disorders in funding allocation. NIMH's new framework for research, the Research Domain Criteria (RDoC), is currently the main document based on which research on mental disorders is conducted. These research frameworks and funding allocations are indicative of research programs that are prioritized or, conversely, undervalued and marginalized. Therefore, they play an important role in my analysis of psychiatry's clinical and scientific vision.

2.2 "A much better job with patients": A history of psychiatry's twin commitments

As psychiatrist Samuel Guze eloquently put it, a fundamental motivation for understanding the nature of psychiatric conditions is not "simply to satisfy one's curiosity and receive greater intellectual stimulation," but "to be able to do a *much better job* with" patients (Guze 1992, 3; my emphasis). Multiple paths can be taken to do "a better job" of improving patients' conditions. Modern psychiatry took the path of developing scientifically valid constructs of mental disorders which can be investigated and measured by scientific tools. Contemporary diagnostic manuals such as the International Classification of Diseases (ICD) published by the World Health Organization (WHO), the DSM published by the American Psychiatric Association (APA), as well as research program guides such as the RDoC published by NIMH, adopt such approaches. Creating valid constructs of mental disorders and investigating their properties are considered important steps in the development of effective clinical interventions and arriving at scientifically objective knowledge about mental disorders. While there is no robust and universally agreed upon notion of effective treatment in psychiatry (Steel and Tekin 2021), the goal, broadly stated, is to enable patients to flourish, by either helping patients fully recover from a mental disorder, arriving at a no-mental-disorder state, or helping them lead an independent and fulfilling life despite the disorder. Thus, psychiatry's twin commitments to developing effective clinical interventions on mental disorders, while also establishing itself as a scientific inquiry, evolved jointly, under the influence of the scientific and cultural zeitgeist of the time. As I explain in Section 3, psychiatry's emphasis on establishing itself as a legitimate form of scientific inquiry that attains the ideal of objectivity has inadvertently led to its shortcomings in clinical contexts.

2.2.1 The DSM, psychoanalysis, and the Freud problem

The primary reason for developing a classification of mental disorders in the United States was to collect statistical information on the prevalence of mental disorders. The 1840 census, conducted by the US Census Office, provided the first formal recording of the frequency of "idiocy/insanity" in the population. Following this, the Association of Medical Superintendents of American Institutions for the Insane was formed in 1844 to develop a classification system for mental disorders created by medical experts—not by the US Census Office. The Association (later the APA) worked with the National Commission on Mental Hygiene (now Mental Health America) to develop a guide for mental hospitals called the Statistical Manual for the Use of Institutions for the Insane (American Psychiatric Association 1952). The Statistical Manual was designed to help administrators of inpatient mental hospitals collect institutional data, not to guide treatment of specific patients. The manual framed the mental disorders it classified as arising from somatic, constitutional, and heredity factors. The Statistical Manual became the definitive taxonomy between World War I and World War II and went through ten editions between 1918 and 1942 (Horwitz 2015a). It offered a standard classification scheme for the psychiatric profession during this era when most psychiatrists practiced in public hospitals and used somatic methods to treat mental disorders (Horwitz 2015a).

An impetus to replace the Statistical Manual emerged during World War II, when psychiatrists became heavily involved in the selection, assessment, and treatment of soldiers and realized the existing descriptions in the manual were a poor fit for the psychiatric casualties of the war. Clinicians increasingly recognized mental disorders often arose because of psychosocial

factors, not merely as a result of somatic processes, and the Statistical
Manual's emphasis on somatic treatments were not always helpful (Horwitz
2015a). In 1943 a committee of American psychiatrists developed a new
classification scheme, Medical 203, and published this in a War Department
technical bulletin. Shortly after World War II, in 1949, the WHO published
the sixth edition of the ICD, which, for the *first* time, included a section on
mental disorders.

Despite efforts to come up with a common classification system useful for
clinical and administrative contexts, by the mid-twentieth century, many
different systems were in use, and there was mounting concern about the
lack of a unifying schema to understand and treat mental disorders (American Psychiatric Association 1952). In response, an APA Committee on
Nomenclature and Statistics developed a system of classification specifically
for use in the United States to standardize the diverse and often inconsistent
usage of different documents listing the criteria for mental disorders. In 1950
the APA Committee undertook a review of Medical 203 by consulting the
members of the APA and the Veterans Administration (VA)—owing to its
continued use of classifications to determine who was fit to serve in war—
and published the first edition of the DSM (DSM-I) in 1952.

The DSM-I had statistical goals: it aimed "to make possible the gathering
of data for future clarification of ideas concerning etiology, pathology,
prognosis, and treatment in mental disorders" (American Psychiatric Association 1952, 9). The APA recognized there were many unknowns about
mental disorders, and the presumption was that as scientific research
advanced, the diagnostic criteria for mental disorders would evolve. This
remains the current vision of the APA. Over time, the etiology underlying
each psychiatric kind would be revealed, making it possible to construct a
classificatory system based on true natural similarities and differences
between various mental disorders. Until then, categories would continue to
be revised to ensure they had "an extensive empirical foundation" and
were useful for "clinical, research, and educational purposes" (American
Psychiatric Association 1994, xxiii).

The DSM-I offered etiological descriptions of mental disorders, i.e.,
explaining mental disorders in relation to their causes, owing largely to the
influence of the psychoanalytic movement spearheaded by Sigmund Freud
that had shaped psychiatry around the world since the early 1900s. Broadly
stated, psychoanalysis develops etiological/causal theories of personality
development, i.e., how childhood experiences and parental relationships
shape the individual (Freud 1896, 1917). It construes the mind as having
conscious layers directly accessible by the individual, as well as unconscious
layers; in this theory, the mental functioning of adults comprises reactions to
(mostly) unrecalled childhood events of a sexual nature (stored in the
unconscious). Psychoanalysts therefore treat mental disorders by investigating the interaction of conscious and unconscious elements in the patient's

mind, using techniques such as dream interpretation, free association, and hypnosis. Over time, psychoanalytic theory gained popularity in clinical and academic areas of psychiatry in the United States, and in 1946, it was officially acknowledged as the leading school of thought by the American Board of Psychiatry.

A notable figure in the promotion of psychoanalytic theory was Adolf Meyer, a neurologist, whose interests shifted to psychiatry as a result of Freud's influence after his move from Switzerland to the United States in 1892 (Houts 2000). Meyer initially believed mental disorder was a biologically specifiable natural disease explained by chemistry and physiology, but he later viewed psychopathology as habit patterns of the person in reaction to emotional states brought about by psychological, social, and biological factors in the circumstances of life.

The DSM-I's description of mental disorders conveyed the psychoanalytic approach. It identified two major groups of mental disorders, focusing on their etiology, i.e., causal mechanisms. The first group comprised "those in which there is disturbance of mental function resulting from...a primary impairment of the function of the brain, generally owing to diffuse impairment of brain tissue," including impairment of intellectual functions, such as memory, orientation, and judgment, and shallowness of affect. These brain dysfunction-based conditions could be the *only* mental disturbance present, or they could be associated with *additional conditions* of the second group of mental disorders. These were characterized as individuals' "reactions" to environmental stressors and were seen as "the result of a more general difficulty in *adaptation* of the *individual*, and...any associated brain function disturbance is secondary to the psychiatric disorder" (American Psychiatric Association 1952, 9; my emphasis). This second group was framed as the maladjustment model of mental disorders. It included: 1) affective disorders, characterized by severe mood disturbance and alterations in thought and behavior; 2) schizophrenic reactions, characterized by fundamental disturbances in reality relationships and concept formations; and 3) paranoid reactions, characterized by persistent delusions. Disorders in this group were descriptively classified as "psychotic," "neurotic," or "behavioral," emphasizing mental disorders as adaptive reactions to the states of affairs in a person's life, not autonomous entities that develop independently from the person. These reactions are not necessarily related in severity to the degree of the organic brain syndrome and are "*as much determined by inherent personality patterns, the social setting, and the stresses of interpersonal relations* as by the precipitating organic impairment" (American Psychiatric Association 1952, 9; my emphasis).

The DSM-II was published in 1968, and it retained the DSM-I's overall approach by continuing to conceptualize psychopathology using a psychodynamic perspective; changes were minimal (First 2010). Insofar as it was influenced by the psychoanalytic framework, it inherited the DSM-I's theoretical presuppositions about the mind. For example, a major family of disorders in the DSM-I was psychoneurotic disorders:

> The chief characteristic of these disorders is "anxiety" which may be directly felt and expressed, or which may be unconsciously and automatically controlled by the utilization of various psychological defense mechanisms (depression, conversion, displacement, etc.). "Anxiety" in psychoneurotic disorders is a danger signal felt and perceived by the conscious portion of the personality. It is produced by a threat from within the personality (e.g., by supercharged repressed emotions, including such aggressive impulses as hostility and resentment), with or without stimulation from such external situations as loss of love, loss of prestige, or threat of injury.
>
> (American Psychiatric Association 1952, 31–2; see also Cooper and Blashfield 2016; Horwitz 2015b)

The psychoanalytic influence is plain in this excerpt: the focus is on theoretical entities, such as the unconscious, impulses, and attempts to connect these to the conscious.

Even though the concept of the individual was not fully developed and did not reflect the sophisticated complexity of the self, both the DSM-I and the DSM-II used terms like "person" or "personality" in making sense of mental disorders. Following the tradition of psychoanalysis, there was an effort to center mental disorders in relation to the individuals experiencing them. Note, however, that the psychoanalytic conception of the individual is largely a theoretical construct, not grounded on an empirically informed notion of the self. In this construct, individuals are guided by the unconscious and conscious forces of the mind, and the goal of psychoanalysis is to sort out the tensions emerging within. Multiple assumptions are made about how personality is shaped by "repressed emotions" or "psychological defense mechanisms." The consideration of social relationships in personality development is limited to how they affect the individual's unconscious and conscious mind.

Even though Freud considered psychoanalysis to be a scientific inquiry into the mind, he and other proponents did not use empirical methods to investigate phenomena but focused on what they observed in their patients in their private practice. Thus, psychoanalysis falls short of a scientific approach to the self—the subject of mental disorder. In fact, its lack of empirical rigor, or the "unfalsifiability" of its claims, in the words of Karl Popper, led to criticism of psychoanalytic theory in philosophical and scientific circles at the time (Popper 1959). For Popper, even though Freudian analysts suggested their theories about psychopathology were confirmed by their clinical observations, confirmations are not good standards for the scientific credibility of a view; in fact, it is easy to obtain confirmations or verifications if we look for them. Instead, he proposed that falsifiability should be looked for when seeking to demarcate science from pseudoscience; to be ranked as "scientific," statements or systems of statements must be capable of conflicting with possible or conceivable observations. Psychoanalysis, under this standard, fails the test of falsifiability. Similarly, Adolf Grünbaum questioned the empirical evidence base for Freud's claims that human behavior is significantly influenced by unconscious thoughts (Grünbaum 1984). Furthermore, as I later explain, the psychoanalytic approach to the individual portrayed in the DSM-I and the DSM-II led to what can be called the *Freud problem* in contemporary scientific psychiatry, in that there is an over-association of concepts like the self or person with psychoanalysis and a connected reluctance to engage with the self in the context of psychiatry because psychoanalysis is believed to be unscientific.

Psychoanalytic approaches to mental disorders centering on the concept of the individual proposed by the DSM-I and DSM-II were favored by the government agencies that provided research funding for mental disorders. In 1947 the US Public Health Service Division of Mental Hygiene awarded the first mental health research grant, Basic Nature of the Learning Process, to Dr. Winthrop N. Kellogg of Indiana University, a comparative psychologist. His project aimed to show how environmental factors affect learning and cognitive development. It emphasized that the development of the person involves both nature and nurture. Similarly, in 1961 the Action for Mental Health Report provided an assessment of mental health conditions of individuals and resources for their care in the United States, with the goal of arriving at a national program to meet the needs of the mentally ill. In 1963, under the leadership of President John F. Kennedy, Congress passed the Mental Retardation Facilities and Community Mental Health Centers Construction Act, under which the National Institute of Mental Health assumed responsibility for monitoring community mental health centers' programs. The priority of these NIMH-funded programs was to offer person-level care to individuals with mental disorders in the community. Shortly thereafter, in 1964, President Lyndon B. Johnson passed what is often referred to as the "War on Poverty" legislation; under his direction, NIMH funded several studies on the socioeconomic and environmental factors affecting the development of mental illness, with a special focus on crime, urban discord, and minority groups' mental health (National Institute of Mental Health 2024). With the shift in the DSM's focus over time, the funding priorities also shifted away from people and their communities to biological markers of mental disorders.

2.2.2 Psychoanalysis and its critics, the path to behaviorism, and the medical model

Psychoanalytic approaches to mental disorders lost much of their popularity in the 1960s, owing to a perfect storm of factors, including concerns about the scientific legitimacy of psychoanalysis, the increasing popularity of alternative theories of the mind such as behaviorism, and the rise of biological approaches to psychiatry that promoted a medical model of mental disorders. Critics targeted the unscientific nature of the diagnostic categories in the DSM-I and the DSM-II, arguing the theoretical assumptions about the functioning of the mind postulated by psychoanalysis do not rely on empirical evidence, and this impedes progress towards scientific objectivity. Simply stated, mental disorder categories lacked scientific validity (Beck 1962; Katz et al. 1968; Schwartz and Wiggins 1987a, 1987b), and psychiatrists were unable to demarcate even the fundamental conditions such as schizophrenia or manic depression. A condition one clinician called "schizophrenia" could be called "manic depression" by others (Robins and Guze 1970; First et al. 2004). The lack of reliability and objectivity were consequences of a diagnostic system that relied on theoretical presuppositions instead of observable features of psychopathology. The combination of the lack of formal criteria for diagnosis and unfalsifiable theoretical assumptions in each definition led clinicians to rely on their subjective intuitions about what they were treating. Large-scale clinical trials were impossible, as the lack of reliable diagnostic categories made it impossible for multiple researchers to replicate the findings (Horwitz 2015a).

Problems with the nature of the diagnostic categories led to a decline in psychiatrists' credibility in the profession, and they were challenged by clinical psychologists and social workers who considered themselves equally qualified to provide care for individuals with mental disorders. The boundaries of the conditions specified in the DSM-I and DSM-II were so broad that they overlapped with the processes emphasized in these other disciplines. Medical training, therefore, seemed irrelevant for understanding the kinds of psychodynamic processes the diagnostic manuals assumed were behind the development of mental illnesses. There was "nothing explicitly *psychiatric* about the assumptions of the first two DSMs: nonmedical and medical professionals alike could diagnose and manage most of the entities that they defined" (Horwitz 2015a). This motivated psychiatry to actively distance itself from disciplines like psychology and rebrand itself as a branch of medicine.

There was also increased criticism of psychoanalysis as a scientific approach to the mind. Behaviorism was gaining traction as an alternative, with an emphasis on measuring behavior to understand the mind, rather than concentrating on unobservable dimensions like the unconscious. Emerging as a school of thought in the 1920s, the behaviorist movement pioneered by John B. Watson, Ivan Pavlov, and B.F. Skinner rejected all the mentalistic concepts of psychoanalysis, such as the unconscious. Behaviorism was influential in attempts to ground diagnostic categories on observable signs and symptoms rather than mental phenomena.

With the competition between behaviorism and psychoanalysis and the declining credibility of psychoanalysis, the medical model of mental disorders started to gain traction. The model was promoted by a group of biologically oriented researchers, who emphasized the need for careful definitions of each mental disorder and objected to the theoretical assumptions underlying the DSM-I and DSM-II definitions. For example, Samuel Guze, a staunch defender of applying the medical model to mental disorders, was among the leading critics of the DSM's psychoanalytic orientation (Guze 1978, 1992). In the medical model, psychiatry was considered a branch of medicine devoted to the study and treatment of psychopathology, defined as disorders in mental and psychological functions. Thus, it used the jargon of general medicine, such as "diagnosis," "differential diagnosis," "etiology," "pathogenesis," "treatment," and "epidemiology," in approaching the diagnosis and treatment of mental disorders. Mental disorders were thought to be "caused by distinctive pathophysiological processes in the brain" that emerge "as collections of behavioral symptoms and signs that occur together and unfold in characteristic ways" (Murphy 2011, 425). If the properties of mental disorders can be delineated in reference to behavioral and neurobiological markers, reliable generalizations can be made about their course, and effective interventions can be developed to address populations with mental disorders—not just a few individuals. The model assumed understanding the brain through advances in neurobiology was pivotal to understanding mental disorders and creating suitable interventions (Guze 1978, 1992). Accordingly, as more was learned about the body, i.e., its development, structure, and function, from the integrative activity of the whole body to its cellular and molecular processes, it would become increasingly feasible to understand, treat, and prevent disease.

At the time, there was a connected assumption that different drugs target distinct mental disorders, and the proponents of the medical model advocated the development of a more precise diagnostic system than that provided by the DSM-I and the DSM-II. If mental disorders could be classified in relation to the behaviors that are displayed, which would be measurable, then the underlying mechanisms for that behavior could be investigated. Thus, the behavioristic framework of the mind was incorporated into the medical model. Proponents like Guze recognized that many disciplines, such as psychology, social work, theology, and law, are interested in understanding mental disorders. Nevertheless, in their view, "*only* psychiatry, as a medical specialty, offers the basis for a comprehensive approach" to mental disorders because only psychiatry directly engages with their biological underpinnings (Guze 1992, 4; my emphasis).

Increased interest in the medical model shaped medical education as well. Notably, in 1969, Eliot Slater and Martin Roth published a textbook applying the medical model to psychiatry. This book remains a classic in medical education and training in psychiatry. Holding physics as the paradigmatic example of science, Slater and Roth endorsed the virtues of biological medicine over sociology as the basis of psychiatric science, arguing, "Our knowledge of medicine gives us information about individuals;

sociological knowledge gives us information only about groups, from which deductions about the individual are notoriously subject to error" (Slater and Roth 1969, 250–251). In their view, an "excessive preoccupation with individuals is heuristically sterile," and in experimental biology, "individual variation is classifiable, statistically, as error" (Slater and Roth 1969, 251). In other words, they encouraged scientists to focus on the observable and generalizable features of mental disorders from a purely biological perspective, not to focus on the individuals encountering them. In this view, the objectivity of psychiatry was only attainable through observable and generalizable features, and a focus on individuals would detract from this ideal.

Finally, adding to critics' concerns, psychiatric diagnoses differed significantly between Europe and the United States (Cooper et al. 1969) because of discrepancies in the mental disorder taxonomies provided by the ICD-6, ICD-7, and DSM-I. The WHO, the creator of the ICD, provided a comprehensive review of diagnostic issues, emphasizing the need for explicit definitions of disorders as a means of promoting reliable clinical diagnoses and calling for the individuation of a condition with the same diagnosis across different theoretical and practical settings. Spearheaded by Erwin Stengel, the review emphasized the value of the diagnostic classification system for the scientific status of psychiatry as a discipline. The target of inquiry, mental disorder, should be consistent throughout the world. In other words, the characteristics of an individual's mental disorder (e.g., schizophrenia) should be the same in the United States and the United Kingdom. A series of diagnostic revisions followed this review, leading to the publication of the DSM-III (and ICD-8).

2.2.3 The DSM-III publication process

The drive to revise the DSM culminated in a turn to philosophical debates about the nature of scientific inquiry to arrive at diagnostic categories that could facilitate scientific research (e.g., Hempel 1961; Popper 1959).[2] Carl Hempel, an established philosopher of science, was invited to give a lecture at the APA's 1959 meeting on scientific taxonomies. In his lecture, he addressed psychiatrists' worries about the validity and reliability of mental disorder classifications in the DSM and highlighted the importance of using "operationalism" to increase the validity and reliability of scientific classifications, thereby enhancing psychiatry's scientific credibility (Hempel 1961, cited in Sadler et al. 1994).

Operationalism is a scientific method spearheaded by physicist Percy Williams Bridgman, who argued a physical theory is understood primarily by which laboratory procedures scientists perform to test its predictions. He found scientific concepts in physics were abstract and unclear and therefore not easily accessible for scientific research. He attempted to redefine unobservable entities by highlighting the physical and mental operations used to measure them (Bridgman 1938; Chang 2019). In other words, operationalism sets out to characterize a complex scientific phenomenon with a focus on its most salient features in a way that lends itself to scientific measurement and analysis. Consider an example from psychology. A psychological variable, such as anger, is not immediately obvious or tractable. Psychologists use operationalism to calculate the behavioral or physiological features of "anger," such as loudness of voice or blood pressure. Such indirect measures are the operational definitions of anger. For a definition of a complex phenomenon to be operational, the steps followed to develop the definitions must be repeatable by anyone, or at least by the peers of the scientist. This ensures the validity of the descriptions in that they are responsive to the facts of the world and appear in different contexts.

In the following passage from his presentation to the psychiatrists at the APA meeting, Hempel is clearly promoting Bridgeman's operationalism:

> An operational definition for a given term is conceived as providing objective criteria by means of which any scientific investigator can decide, for any particular case, whether the term does or does not apply.... Most diagnostic procedures used in medicine are based on the operational criteria of application for corresponding diagnostic categories.
>
> (Hempel 1961, cited in Sadler et al. 1994, 319)

Note that Hempel, synching with the proponents of the medical model, urges psychiatrists to develop operational definitions in psychiatry, as in other areas of medicine. He asks psychiatrists to take the concept of operation in a "liberal" sense, suggesting that the:

> "mere observation of an object ... must be allowed to count as an operation, for the criteria of application for a term may well be specified by reference to certain characteristics which can be ascertained without any testing procedure more complicated than direct observation."
>
> (Hempel 1961, cited in Sadler et al. 1994, 320)

In a psychiatric context, then, operational definitions must depict the properties of mental disorders which are directly observable by different observers, thereby warranting a consistent intersubjective agreement on their descriptions. Observations of behavior (expressed in the form of symptoms and signs) are the obvious measures for mental disorders. Operational descriptions serve two purposes in Hempel's image of science:

> [T]he vocabulary of science has two basic functions: first, to permit an adequate *description* of the things and events that are the objects of scientific investigation; second, to permit the establishment of general laws or theories by means of which particular events may be *explained*

and *predicted* and thus *scientifically understood*; for to understand a phenomenon scientifically is to show that it occurs in accordance with general laws or theoretical principles.

(Hempel 1961, cited in Sadler et al. 1994, 317; emphasis in original)

For psychiatry to establish itself as a science, Hempel says psychiatrists should use operational descriptions, as they will eventually lend themselves to the development of laws and theories through which we can explain and predict mental disorders. He criticizes the psychoanalytic framework used in the DSM-I and DSM-II, taking exception to the lack of operational descriptions in their characterization of mental disorders. One example is the DMS-I's "conversion reaction," whereby anxiety is "converted into functional symptoms in organs or parts of the body, usually those that are mainly under voluntary control" (American Psychiatric Association 1952, 32–33). Hempel notes:

Clearly, several of the terms used in this passage refer neither to directly observable phenomena, such as overt behavior, nor to responses that can be elicited by suitable stimuli, but rather to theoretically assumed psychodynamic factors. Those terms have a distinct meaning and function only in the context of corresponding theory; just as the terms *gravitational field, gravitational potential,* and so on have a definite meaning and function only in the context of a corresponding theory of gravitation.

(Hempel 1961, cited in Sadler et al. 1994, 318; emphasis in original)

Note that Hempel is encouraging both the development of descriptions that can be observable, such as behavior, and the distancing of such terms from existing theoretical frameworks. The concept of the "unconscious," for example, is only meaningful when we take psychodynamic theory as the background. For Hempel, operationalism could increase the reliability of the mental disorder categories by allowing different clinicians to individuate the same phenomena for the same mental disorder, thus securing their objectivity. Hempel says:

One of the main objections to various types of contemporary psychodynamic theories, for example, is that their central concepts lack clear and uniform criteria of application, and that, as a consequence, there are no definite and unequivocal ways of putting the theories to a test by applying them to concrete cases. ... For just this reason, the operational criteria of application for psychological terms are usually formulated by reference to publicly observable aspects of the behavior a subject shows in response to a specified publicly observable stimulus situation, and this does indeed seem to be the most satisfactory way of meeting the demands of scientific objectivity.

(Hempel 1961, cited in Sadler et al. 1994, 318–321)

In Hempel's view, then, for psychiatry to be scientific, it must start with operational descriptions validating the phenomenon under scrutiny; this is the route to scientific objectivity.

Following Hempel's talk at the APA, psychiatrists at Washington University in St. Louis developed a set of diagnostic criteria that aligned with the Hempelian operationalist approach. John Feighner, Eli Robins, Samuel Guze, and George Winokur had been working together on developing a medical model of psychiatric diagnosis since the late 1950s. In a 1972 paper, they proposed criteria for diagnosing 14 psychiatric disorders, including primary affective disorders (such as depression), schizophrenia, anxiety neurosis, and antisocial personality disorder. The criteria for diagnoses were based on studies of outpatients and inpatients, on family studies, and on follow-up studies, and the categories were validated by clinicians. The Feighner criteria (named after the first author of the paper) were conceived to be "the most efficient currently available; however, it is expected that the criteria be tested and not be considered a final, closed system" (Feighner et al. 1972). In other words, the criteria would change as various illnesses were further studied by different groups of scientists. However, for the time being, the criteria provided a framework for the comparison of data gathered in different centers and promoted communication between investigators (Bluhm 2017).

One of the influential figures in the process was Robert Spitzer, whose work focused on the measurement of psychopathology and the development of survey instruments and structured interviews. In 1978 he led the expansion of the Feighner criteria into the Research Diagnostic Criteria and its companion, the Schedule for Affective Disorders and Schizophrenia. Spitzer was later appointed to oversee the revision of the DSM-III (1980). Most of the mental disorder criteria in the DSM-III were based on the Research Diagnostic Criteria. The Feighner criteria also shaped the WHO's ICD manual. Some argue the Feighner criteria instigated "a paradigm shift that has had profound effects on the course of American and, ultimately, world psychiatry" (Kendler et al. 2010), simply because for the first time in the history of psychiatry, mental disorders were categorized on the basis of their observable features as opposed to theoretical assumptions about what kinds of things mental disorders are.

2.3 Contemporary framework for mental disorders

The DSM-III made multiple changes to the DSM framework, most of which remain the same in the most recent revision, the DSM-5-TR. The DSM-III operationalized the diagnostic criteria for every mental disorder in the face of opposition from the psychoanalytic community. One of its key attributes was the specification of symptoms and signs, following Hempel's above-mentioned recommendation that mental disorders be described through "publicly observable aspects of the behavior of a subject." Consequently, it was consistent across the mental health-care community and widely accepted by researchers and clinicians in the USA and internationally. A new diagnosis championed by Dr. Spitzer as part of the DSM-III process was post-traumatic stress disorder, added in the context of increased recognition of the psychological wounds of combat exposure among soldiers returning from the Vietnam War. As this example suggests, it is perhaps best to think of the DSM as a "work-in-progress," as the knowledge on mental disorders is incomplete, complex, and dynamic, making it open to updates and changes in light of the most recent scientific work.

With the DSM-III and all following DSMs including the current one, the emphasis shifted from theoretical explanations of the causes of mental disorders to the observable and measurable features of psychopathology. Each diagnostic category, for example, major depression, is operationalized through a list of observable behaviors clustered as symptoms (observed and reported by the patient) and signs (observed and reported by others). In this schema, mental disorders are described according to physical or psychological experiences that correspond to a set of behaviors, observable by the person experiencing them and verifiable by an observer. Take insomnia. An individual can report this experience, and it can be corroborated by an observer. Some observable features are psychological, for example, feelings of sadness, and others are physical, for example, palpitation and disturbances of vegetative functions (e.g., appetite loss, weight gain) (American Psychiatric Association 2013).

The DSM uses polythetic criteria sets, as opposed to monothetic criteria sets, to determine the boundaries of a disorder category. Monothetic classifications are based on the characteristics that are both necessary and sufficient for the identification of members of a class; each member must have at least one property shared with all members. In polythetic classifications, each member of a class shares a large proportion of its properties with other members, but all members do not necessarily share any one property (Guze 1978; Sokal 1974). For instance, according to the criteria for depression in the DSM-5, at least five symptoms have to be present during a two-week period and must represent a change from the patient's previous functioning. Either "depressed mood" or "diminished interest in and pleasure from daily activities" must be among the five. Additional symptoms include a combination of the following: significant weight loss or gain, insomnia or hypersomnia, psychomotor agitation, fatigue or loss of energy, feelings of worthlessness or inappropriate guilt, diminished ability to think or concentrate, indecisiveness, recurrent thoughts of death, and suicidal ideation (American Psychiatric Association 2013, 125).

Finally, the DSM diagnostic criteria include clauses that attempt to prevent misdiagnosis. If the symptoms are accounted for by the direct physiological effects of a substance or by a general medical condition, a depression diagnosis cannot be made. Symptom- (observed by the patient) and sign-

(observed by others) based descriptions of mental disorders are demonstrations of the DSM's operationalism. Still in use, they are thought to advance scientific and clinical utility, as they promote valid and reliable scientific categories (American Psychiatric Association 1994, xv; 2013, xli). A diagnostic category of depression based on symptoms and signs is believed to have validity because the diagnosed individual exhibits behaviors or feelings that are typical of depression (insomnia, loss of interest in previously enjoyable activities, etc.). It also has reliability because the same set of observable behaviors will be individuated as the same mental disorder regardless of the context. Thus, the symptom- and sign-based approach, by simplifying a complex target such as mental disorders, helps validate the mental disorder constructs by identifying common signs and symptoms and creates reliable categories that can be used across settings.

A focus on the observable features of mental disorders also served the interests of the medical model. Based on the observable features, further research into the genetic and neural underpinnings of mental disorders could be generated by, say, performing imaging studies on the brains of depressed individuals suffering from insomnia. In fact, the DSM-5 offers a definition of mental disorder that is shaped by the medical model:

> A mental disorder is a syndrome characterized by clinically significant disturbance in an individual's cognition, emotion regulation, or behavior that reflects a dysfunction in the psychological, biological, or development processes underlying mental functioning. Mental disorders are usually associated with significant distress or disability in social, occupational, or other important activities. An expectable or culturally approved response to a common stressor or loss, such as the death of a loved one, is not a mental disorder. Socially deviant behavior (e.g., political, religious, or sexual) and conflicts that are primarily between the individual and society are not mental disorders unless the deviance or conflict results from a dysfunction in the individual, as described above.
> (American Psychiatric Association 2013)

The medical model is evident here, as the emphasis is on an "underlying dysfunction," purportedly the reason for mental disorders. Contemporary brain disease models of mental disorders are other good examples of the medical model insofar as they focus on neurobiological or cellular-level frameworks to explain the mechanisms underlying disorders and pave the way for mostly medical interventions. Psychopharmacology, i.e., treatment of mental disorders with medications, is based on the medical model, as medications are assumed to target and correct physiological problems underlying mental disorders. In this sense, research priorities include basic science research, research on neurobiological mechanisms for mental disorders, development of drugs targeting these mechanisms, and so on.

Beyond the DSM revisions, the shift to symptom- and sign-based models of mental disorders was apparent in NIMH's funding priorities to projects studying cellular-level frameworks. For example, in 1970, NIMH researcher Dr. Julius Axelrod won the Nobel Prize for research on the chemistry of nerve transmission. He found an enzyme that stops the action of the neurotransmitter noradrenaline—a critical target of many antidepressant drugs—in the synapse. Similarly, in a major development in the treatment of bipolar disorder, in 1970, the US Food and Drug Administration approved the use of lithium as a treatment for mania, leading to sharp drops in inpatient days and suicides among people with bipolar disorder (National Institute of Mental Health 2024).

Advances continued in the 1980s with the development of a new method of measuring brain function that contributed to the basic understanding and diagnosis of brain diseases, i.e., positron emission tomography (PET) scanning. This was the first imaging technology to permit scientists to "observe" and obtain visual images of the living, functioning brain. This increased the optimism that neuroscience would eventually lead to the discovery of treatments for all mental disorders. The 1990s were declared the "decade of the brain," and NIMH established the Human Brain Project to develop, through cutting-edge imaging, computer, and network technologies, a comprehensive neuroscience database accessible via an international computer network (National Institute of Mental Health 2024).

During the late 1990s and into the new century, NIMH dedicated even more resources to neuroscientific research. A significant step in this direction was the establishment of the Basic and Clinical Neuroscience Research Division. In 2000, Eric Kandel and Paul Greengard, each of whom had received NIMH support for more than three decades, shared the Nobel Prize. Kandel received the prize for his work on the functional modification of synapses in the brain. He established that the formation of memories is a consequence of short- and long-term changes in the biochemistry of nerve cells. Greengard was recognized for his discovery that dopamine and several other transmitters can alter the functional state of neuronal proteins. The same year, Nancy Andreasen, also a NIMH grantee, received the National Medal of Science for her work in schizophrenia and for joining behavioral science with neuroscience and neuroimaging (National Institute of Mental Health 2018). In 2008 NIMH implemented a new Strategic Plan to promote discovery in the brain and behavioral sciences to fuel research on the causes, mechanisms, and trajectories of mental disorders to determine when, where, and how to intervene in mental disorders at the cellular level.

Adding to these developments, in 2010 NIMH launched the Research Domain Criteria (RDoC) initiative aimed at developing, for research purposes, new ways of classifying mental disorders based on behavioral dimensions and neurobiological measures. The goal of the RDoC is to create a new conceptual framework for psychiatric research identifying domains of functioning that can be analyzed at several levels, thereby integrating resources from various basic sciences, especially neuroscience, and cognitive science. Until this time, the DSM was used to guide research on mental disorders, in addition to its primary role in diagnostic, treatment, and policy contexts. After the RDoC was created, however, NIMH declared the DSM unsuitable for research purposes (Insel 2013; Insel and Lieberman 2013). The argument was that its categories were no longer appropriate because they lacked validity; a diagnostic system that aims to scrutinize mental illness should more directly reflect modern brain science, as "mental illness will be best understood as disorders of brain structure and function that implicate specific domains of cognition, emotion, and behavior" (Insel and Lieberman 2013).

NIMH's RDoC program does not currently fund research projects unless they explicitly analyze the neurobiology of mental disorder, and it encourages research programs seeking pharmaceuticals to target and rebalance neurobiological breakdown in the brain (Vaidyanathan 2016). However, an exclusive focus on neurobiology discourages alternative initiatives; in the case of substance use disorders, for example, it precludes research into the relationship between homelessness and substance use or intervention strategies involving housing programs for the homeless. Some critics of NIMH's approach have suggested emphasizing the primacy of neuroscientific research in psychopathology continues an unfortunate trend that ignores the crucial role of the phenomenology of mental illness (Graham and Flanagan 2013). Others are concerned that the RDoC lacks suitable attention to relational problems, social processes, and cultural contexts (Hoffman and Zachar 2017). Nonetheless, ongoing research funding indicates a continued emphasis on the brain. Between 2005 and 2014, there was a significant increase in the funding for NIMH's Division of Neuroscience and Basic Behavioral Science (DNBBS), while the funding for the Division of Translational Research went down. In addition, the amount allotted for DNBBS was more than double that for the Division of Services and Intervention Research (Insel 2015).

Let's take stock. As the historical overview demonstrates, psychiatry's twin commitments, first, to develop effective clinical interventions that aid flourishing, and second, to establish itself as a legitimate scientific inquiry, led the DSM to shift to an operational framework for mental disorders in which mental disorders are characterized through their observable features, mostly the behavior of the individual. This was considered a necessary step to increase the validity and reliability of psychiatric diagnoses, thereby enhancing psychiatry's objectivity and scientific credibility. Once mental disorders were operationally defined, it was assumed their underlying causal mechanisms and laws would be revealed through more scientific research. This change was also aligned with the fundamental commitments of the medical model; it was assumed that as more was uncovered about the physiology of the brain, better interventions would be developed. Unfortunately, however, the pursuit of uncovering brain physiology to arrive at better interventions in mental disorders has not fully paid off. While significant advances have been made in unraveling the inner workings of the brain, these advances have not translated into advances in mental health care. Mental disorders are still not fully understood, and the needs of those diagnosed with mental disorders are not met, leaving a persistent gap between scientific research on mental disorders and the clinical needs of those diagnosed with mental illness.

Today, even the promoters of the medical model understand advances in biomedicine and neuroscience are not mirrored by advances in meeting the needs of those diagnosed with mental disorders. Biology alone is insufficient to meet the needs of a growing number of patients, and neuroscience is not here to save psychiatry (Insel 2022). In addition, in the words of the former director of NIMH, Steven Hyman, the "drug revolution stalled" (Hyman 2012). More drug companies are leaving the field. They are no longer developing new psychotropic medications primarily because it is no longer profitable. A limit has been reached in developing medications that help people, and there is increased recognition that they do not consistently help everyone. Moreover, to the extent that they help, they come with so many side effects that individuals are reluctant to take them. Fifty years later, it is safe to suggest the medical model has not delivered what it promised. Contemporary psychiatry is in crisis, and this is harming individuals whose lives are touched by mental disorder.

My contention is that psychiatry's clinical aspirations have not been met because of the way mental disorders are construed. Patients are understood as biological organisms whose mental disorders are expressed through their behavior. Their social, cognitive, narrative, and cultural dimensions are acknowledged, but not truly explored. Efforts to be more scientific may have increased, but the medical model is not tailored to fit the goal of inquiry in psychiatry—an engagement with the cognitive, social, and cultural complexity of the subject who encounters mental disorder. Thus, the attempts to be more scientifically rigorous through operationalism and the medical model have resulted in twin failures.

2.4 Psychiatry's twin failures

As discussed above, mental disorders are characterized in the DSM as a list of observable symptoms and signs. Unfortunately, these lists often provide a thin description of an individual's subjective encounter with mental disorder; not only they do not contextualize the "problematic" behaviors in question, they also do not have much room to examine an individual's mental states such as beliefs, desires, expectations, hopes, etc. As we saw in Chapter 1, a scrutiny of the experiences of people diagnosed with a mental disorder suggests mental disorders are more complex than can be delineated by a list of symptoms and signs. For example, in the case of major depression, precisely how the mental disorder is subjectively encountered and how feelings of worthlessness or depressed mood are experienced are contingent on many other dimensions of a person's life, making this experience unique. Mental disorders intimately intersect with individuals' self-related capacities and attitudes, as well as other subjective contingencies, such as their personal identity, race, gender, or socioeconomic status. Thus, considering these factors is important for clinicians who are trying to help patients and for patients who are trying to get better. Consider this point revisiting Dennett's intentional stance, according to which, the best way to make predictions about humans' behavior is by thinking of them as agents who have psychological states such as beliefs, desires, intentions, etc. Even in the typical cases, explaining and predicting human behavior without adopting an intentional stance is extremely hard: the design and physical stances fall short of fathoming the complexity of human cognition to provide sufficient explanations of behavior. Yet mental states such as intentions are not as "observable" as an operationalist might want them to be: while they can be revealed in self-reports—assuming individuals themselves are aware of their own mental states—it is hard to detect intentions from a third-person or intersubjective standpoint. Attributing intentionality does explain some human behavior well, however. Consider individuals with schizophrenia diagnoses; from a third-person standpoint, their apparent withdrawal can be described as unwillingness to engage in social interaction, as is articulated in the DSM. Yet engaging with individuals with this diagnosis might reveal that they want to or intend to socialize but are unable to do so. In this example, attributing mental states to the individual does important explanatory work which is missed if we focus only on intersubjectively observable behavior.

Thus, the DSM's scientific aspirations have led to twin failures. On the one hand, the complexity of the self who is the subject of mental disorders is sidestepped, owing to an almost exclusive focus on behavior. On the other hand, patients, as subjects who have a direct encounter with mental disorder, have never been considered knowledge generators in psychiatry. Debates in psychiatry have largely ignored the plausibility of identifying the self as a target of scientific inquiry and undermined the value of patients' testimonies in building knowledge on mental disorders. Let's examine these twin failures in turn.

2.4.1 Hyponarrativity and the missing self in the DSM

The DSM descriptions of mental disorders ignore the complexity of the self who is subject to mental disorder. I take the self to be a dynamic, complex, and multi-dimensional mechanism with a degree of agential capacity and autonomy. As I discussed in Chapter 1, the experience of a mental disorder involves the complex mechanism of the self, and the ability to create an effective intervention (clinical or other) is enhanced when the full complexity of the self is taken as a starting point. The fundamental problem with the DSM's symptom- and sign-focused descriptions of mental disorder is their "hyponarrativity" (Sadler 2005), i.e., the use of decontextualized behaviors to describe mental disorders. When the focus is on a set of behaviors isolated from the integrated complexity of the self who encounters a mental disorder, the result is a caricature of a person with mental disorder, not an integrated and resourceful description.

The hyponarrativity of the DSM descriptions can best be articulated in contrast to the hyper-narrativity or the richness of the self. Mental disorders are intimately tied to the identity-constituting features of the self and to the way individuals regard themselves. Identity-constituting features of the self are those that characterize a person and distinguish one person from another. These include physical features, social relationships, personal histories, and the way individuals regard all these features in their self-narratives, i.e., the stories they tell about themselves. For example, an individual's developmental history, future life trajectories, biological and environmental risk factors, interpersonal relationships, race, gender, socioeconomic status, immigration status, etc. are combined to make them who they are and how they are characterized (Schechtman 1997). We might characterize an individual as a "single mother who immigrated to the US from Argentina when she was 20" to describe who this person is. But characterization also depends on why we are telling her life story in the first place. In the context of finding strategies that will help individuals with mental disorders flourish, thinking of mental disorders in relation to the identity-constituting dimensions of the self is important, as it may provide multiple resources for both the clinician and the patient.

However, such features of the self are not taken into consideration in the DSM's mental disorder categories. An individual's behavior is often considered in isolation from the overall self. In the case of the depressed individual, we may learn about low mood or increased appetite, but we do not hear about the interpersonal context that may have given rise to the low mood, or a physical change that may have resulted in the increased appetite. In other words, categories provide a hyponarrative description of the experiences of the individual who is subject to mental disorder. They abstract or bracket the self-related aspects of the encounter. Phenomena that describe a particular person's experience, individual circumstances that play a role in the emergence or aggravation of the condition, and the unique life story that scaffolds the mental disorder are not included in the diagnostic category. This sidelining is deemed necessary for the scientific investigability of mental disorders, because the features of the self are not considered as readily measurable or generalizable across patients. A pervasive assumption in the DSM is that the goal of taxonomizing mental disorders is to find common features across patients and leave aside the subjective features of an individual's particular encounter. By saying little about how the illness experience is integrated into the patient's life as a whole, the DSM criteria, in practice, are "nothing more than a repertoire of behavior" (Cohen 2003).

In addition, the DSM presents the signs and symptoms of a mental disorder as if they unfold autonomously, independent from the subject who is encountering them or the social and cultural context in which they are embedded. Even factors like an individual's stage of life, whether youth or mid-life or old age, are not a part of mental disorder characterizations, even though life stages have an impact on the way an individual encounters a mental disorder. It matters whether the individual with anorexia is a teenager or a 65-year-old, if we want to find a strategy to help them. In short, the descriptions of mental disorders are devoid of the complex narratives that are almost always part of an individual's encounter with a mental disorder. There is little room, as Sadler puts it, for the life narratives that contribute to the nature and course of a patient's mental disorder: "To diagnose a person by means of the DSMs is to unveil very little of her biography" (Sadler 2005, 177). By the person's "biography," he means what is important to them, how they came to be who they are, which people or events had an important influence on them, how the chronological unfolding of their life has shaped their present and will shape their future, and how the experience of illness interacts with these aspects of their life. The finer aspects of their life experiences are not included in the DSM:

> Hyponarrativity loses the intimate interplay of environmental event, individual response, and historical unfolding that characterize important clinical information such as the personal meaning of events, development of the personality, and sensitivity to environmental and interpersonal context. The DSMs' descriptions of mental disorders have no plot line, no particularized conflicts with unique others, no climax, no denouement. To the degree that characters do appear in a DSM category ... they are empty-shell abstractions of people—the exploitees of the narcissistic, the idealized and devalued of the borderline, the beleaguered recipient of erotomanic preoccupations.
>
> (Sadler 2005, 177)

Note that the DSM does not instruct the clinician to "undermine the patient's story." Rather, the assumption seems to be that the clinician will engage with the self-related properties in clinical settings. Several statements in the introduction and throughout the DSM indicate that the diagnostic criteria are not intended to replace a holistic picture of the individual's experience. In fact, some members of the task forces who update the DSM have noted the importance of attending to patients' stories. For instance, Allen Frances, the chair of the DSM-IV task force, warns us not to assume that knowing the diagnosis is the same as knowing the patient (Sadler 2005,

178). The DSM itself recognizes the limitations of the categorical approach (American Psychiatric Association 1994, xxii). The introductions to both the DSM-IV and the DSM-5 emphasize that a categorical approach to classifications works best when all members of a class are homogeneous, when there are clear boundaries, and when the different classes are mutually exclusive. They acknowledge this is not the case in mental disorders. Patients, even if they share a diagnosis, form heterogeneous classes, because each person has a unique encounter, owing to the contingencies of their own lives. They also caution that the categorical system does not imply there are clear boundaries between different mental disorders.

Nonetheless, despite these disclaimers, the emphasis on the symptoms and signs in the definition of mental disorders makes hyponarrativity an important feature of the DSM and is the result of psychiatry's efforts to establish its scientific status by operationalizing mental disorder categories through observables. As will be discussed in detail in Chapter 3, hyponarrativity has epistemic and ethical costs for clinical interventions and for the diagnosed individual, including the way both the individual and society at large make sense of mental disorders. And as will further be discussed in the remainder of the book, there are ways for psychiatry to remain loyal to its scientific aspirations while promoting person-centered clinical care.

2.4.2 Underappreciation and underutilization of first-person reports

The second of psychiatry's twin failures is the underappreciation and underutilization of first- person reports in the development of frameworks for psychiatric diagnoses and psychiatric research. Those who have a direct encounter with a mental disorder have never been considered "experts" who can participate in the knowledge production process in psychiatry. The DSM and RDoC represent the dominant perspectives in scientific psychiatry and are the primary schemas currently used to expand scientific knowledge on mental disorders. As I explain below, they have shared commitments to the concept of expertise; both take experts to be those with recognized training in psychopathology and consider them the primary knowledge generators on mental disorders. Individuals with a diagnosis of mental disorder do not constitute a homogeneous group with shared ideas and commitments. Yet at least some of these individuals, whether implicitly or explicitly, consider themselves experts on their condition. Consider, for example, the growing number of first-person memoirs of mental illness or the explicit claims made by some individuals diagnosed with mental disorders that they are experts by experience (e.g., Frank 1995; Goidsenhoven and Masschelein 2018; Saks 2007). In fact, some patient/consumer/survivor/ex-patient groups requested a seat at the table during the DSM-5 revision process and expressed disappointment at not being considered "experts."

The DSMs have historically been developed and revised in the following manner. The APA selects a task force from the members of the APA. The membership of this task force has evolved over time, but members have mostly been psychiatrists and clinicians. The task force works closely with various working groups who are also mostly psychiatrists and clinicians. The working groups specialize in specific disorders and engage in research and clinical trials to determine how to best classify mental disorders. This collective knowledge generation practice, which can be thought of as an epistemic ritual (Solomon 2015), culminates in the task force's final decisions on the categories of mental disorders. Throughout the history of the DSMs' development, those with a mental disorder have never been included in this process as "subjects" who generate research. A review of the members of the DSM task forces and working groups listed in the introductions of the DSMs—from the DSM-I to the DSM-5—shows patients have never been part of the decision-making process, either as members of the DSM task force or as members of a working group (American Psychiatric Association 1952, 1968, 1980, 1994, 2013). To the extent that they have been part of the DSM research, they have generally remained the "objects" of investigation, for example, recruited for clinical trials. In the DSM-III and the DSM-IV, the APA says it sought the "advice of *experts* in each specific area under consideration" (American Psychiatric Association 1994, xv; my emphasis). "Experts" in the DSMs' language refers to scientifically trained researchers or clinicians with recognized degrees who treat individuals with mental disorders. The introductions to the DSM manuals list the groups consulted in their creation; these include psychiatrists, psychologists, and medical doctors, as well as representatives of psychiatry networks, for example, the members of the Association for Women Psychiatrists. Patients have never been included.

In the DSM-I, the emphasis was on bringing together psychiatrists with different specialties to include representatives of all areas in mental disorder research, as well as various interest groups of specialists in mental health. The foreword to DSM-I also says the US Navy made some revisions to the work (American Psychiatric Association 1952). The military was involved because DSM-I was intended to be a statistical guide to determine fitness to serve in the Korean War (Grinker 2010). In addition, after World War II, many returning American soldiers had combat fatigue and shell shock, relatively mild mental disorders, but the existing conceptions of mental disorders were not responsive to them. To address these pressing needs, the APA decided to expand its categories of mental disorders (Grob 1991). In the further iterations (DSM-II to DSM-5), the status of "expert" was limited to those with clinical training in psychopathology, mostly psychiatrists and psychologists who were members of the APA. In the DSM-II, the military was excluded, but the rest of the group remained the same (American Psychiatric Association 1968). Starting with the DSM-III, while the task force membership remained the same, the APA collected input for the diagnostic criteria, not only from APA-affiliated psychiatrists, but also from scientists and practitioners in other stakeholder organizations, including the American Psychological Association, Association of Women Psychiatrists, and American Psychoanalytic Association (American Psychiatric Association 1980, 1994).

The conception of expertise in the NIMH's RDoC framework is similar to the DSM conception. As it was partly a response to criticism of the DSM's fitness for research purposes, the RDoC offers a framework to investigate mental disorders by integrating different levels of information, including genomics, neural circuits, and behavior. Its goal is the exploration of basic dimensions of human functioning, such as fear circuitry or working memory, rather than disorder or diagnostic discrimination (Tabb 2015), the focus of the DSM. The dimensions span the full range of human cognition and behavior from normal to abnormal and cut across the DSM-5's mental disorder categories; psychiatric investigators present their experiments as targeting fundamental components of mental functioning (or "research domains") based on research from allied sciences, instead of using DSM constructs.

Research domains represent one axis of the proposed matrix, and these are subdivided into more specific "constructs," for example, "reward valuation" or "attachment formation and maintenance." The other axis is "units of analysis," ranging from "genes" to "behavior." The RDoC's self-designated purpose is to translate rapid progress in basic neurobiological and behavioral research to an improved integrative understanding of psychopathology and the development of new and/or optimally matched treatments for mental disorders (Cuthbert 2014). Committed to providing a rigorous framework for research on mental disorders, and critical of the DSM-5 framework, NIMH Director Thomas Insel announced it was time to "re-orient" away from the DSM's symptom-based categories in psychiatric research and said NIMH would fund research using the RDoC framework (Insel 2013).

While there is no explicit discussion of who was consulted to create the RDoC framework, the notion of expertise seems to be reserved for those with technical training in psychopathology. The framework was officially developed by the scientists working for NIMH, and researchers are required to use the RDoC's units of analysis in their applications for NIMH funding. Units of analysis include the following: "circuits," i.e., measurements of brain circuits as studied by neuroimaging techniques and/or other measures validated by animal models or functional neuroimaging; "physiology," i.e., measures such as heart rate and cortisol; "behavior," i.e., behavioral tasks (e.g., a working memory task) or systematic behavioral observations (e.g., a toddler behavioral assessment); and "self-reports," i.e., interview-based scales, self-report questionnaires, or other instruments that may encompass normal-range and/or abnormal aspects of the dimension of the function of interest. All these reflect the assumption that the primary knowledge generators in the investigation of mental functioning are those with research expertise in psychopathology, and patients' perspectives and experiences are simply objects to be studied or synthesized. The problem is that if patients' reports are not considered valid or relevant, researchers may not engage with them and will not make their insights part of the systemic knowledge, even though they may be essential to grasp the phenomenon of interest. In addition, most mental disorders affect the meaning-making system of the individual subject, and understanding their perception of their experiences is essential to address their medical needs and provide care. While unlike the DSM, the RDoC includes an explicit unit of analysis to engage with the self-reports of individuals or patients, thereby highlighting the value of individuals' lived experiences, individuals are considered the *objects* of inquiry, not the *subjects* generating knowledge. An unanalyzed assumption of both the DSM and the RDoC is that patients lack the expertise required for the scientific investigation of mental disorders.

Before the publication of the DSM-5, various groups, including patients, caregivers, mental health activists, advocacy groups, philosophers, and clinicians, invited the APA to involve patients in the revision process by making them members of the task force or a working group. Most calls cited social and political reasons for inclusion. For example, some philosophers and clinicians pushed for the need for the process to be democratic; in their view, participants should include members of the public with a stake in the diagnostic criteria, such as patients, individuals with disabilities, and their families (Sadler and Fulford 2004). Others approached it from the perspective of patient advocacy and emphasized the need "for scientific experts to review their nosological recommendations in light of rigorous consideration of consumer experience and feedback" (Stein and Phillips 2013). This would, for example, mean patients would give feedback on a proposed criterion for a mental disorder category developed by the psychiatrists on the task force. Epistemic and ethical reasons were also cited. Some psychiatrists argued for the value of patients' subjective experiences; this, they said, would help the DSM criteria for mental disorders to be finer-grained and more responsive to the real experiences of patients (Flanagan, Davidson, and Strauss 2010).[3]

The DSM-5 task force showed some sympathy for the social and political reasons, as it acknowledged the potential benefits of patients' inclusion in the DSM creation process. Yet it suggested the time frame was too limited for an elaborate engagement. It further suggested the APA's call for public feedback on the DSM-5 through an online forum was a positive step towards including patient input, insofar as patients are also members of the public. Note that in the DSM-5 task force response, patients' potential contributions were framed as having the same value as those of the general public—the ability of their unique standpoint, as those directly encountering mental disorder, to improve the diagnostic criteria for mental disorders was dismissed. In fact, the DSM-5 task force had epistemic concerns about patient inclusion. They thought the "subjectivity of the data" in patients' reports conflicted with psychiatry's desire to establish itself as an objective form of inquiry (Regier et al. 2010). To explain why patients were not invited to be a part of the DSM-5 revision process, the task force stated the following:

> We recognize that subjecting criteria to patient review may allow DSM-V to draw a more complete and clinically meaningful picture of disorders based on individual experiences ... of patients. ... Integrating objective diagnostic criteria and patient-subjective data may serve to enhance the therapeutic alliance, since it could assist the clinician in better understanding the source of an individual patient's distress, not simply the clinician's preconceived assertions about what a given diagnosis is and is not. By definition, subjectivity is variable from person to person, therefore making it impossible to develop definitive criteria that would apply to every disorder.
>
> (Regier et al. 2010, 309)

Regier and colleagues do not define precisely what they mean by "objective" or "subjective" in the context of the DSM creation, but I offer some possible interpretations in Chapter 6. For now, let me emphasize that following the statement above, the DSM-5 was published without patient input. Patients were not included on the task force or the working groups. Nor were they invited to provide systematic feedback by virtue of their status as patients.

As I discussed in Chapter 1, involving patients in the psychiatric knowledge process is necessary, and not doing so is a missed opportunity. The unknowns of mental disorders are still greater than the knowns, so we have to commit to the practice (rather than the products) of psychiatric research as it unfolds. In addition, engaging patients is the best way to understand their subjective experiences and should be set alongside scientific paradigms tackling subjective experience, such as inquiry in psychology and cognitive science.

If we pay attention to the nature of research in psychiatry, the inclusion of patients in the group of researchers working on mental disorders is necessary for epistemic reasons; patient inclusion in the process will help psychiatry attain scientific objectivity. Psychiatry is an intervention-oriented science; its main goal is the discovery of the scientifically relevant properties of mental disorders that yield successful explanations, reliable predictions, and effective interventions. To discover and then investigate these features, it is necessary to examine not only the clinical and scientific work on mental disorders but also the first-person reports of those experiencing them. Taken together, as I show in Chapter 5, these epistemic resources may help develop interventions, as they may clarify what it is like to have a mental disorder, disclose the underlying causes, and suggest treatment. In addition, they will help advance psychiatry's scientific commitments.

Note the connection between psychiatry's twin failures. The first, hypo-narrativity, is a thin or shallow conception of selfhood, where disorders are defined in terms of observable behaviors. One way to remedy this would be to engage with research in cognitive sciences to better fathom self-related features of mental disorders. Another would be to directly engage with first-person reports of individuals with mental disorders. However, the latter solution is precluded by the second twin failure: self-reports are not used to make sense of mental disorders. Even so, understanding the subjective features of mental disorders requires more than simply giving space to patient reports; in other words, patient reports are necessary to examine self-related features of mental disorders, but these alone are not sufficient to achieve larger understanding; we also need cognitive sciences such as psychology to examine them.

2.5 Conclusion

In this historical chapter, I traced the evolution of psychiatry's twin commitments: to develop effective clinical interventions and to establish itself as a scientific discipline. I argued that the effort to enhance its scientific status has resulted in the undermining of its clinical goals because it has involved sidestepping the self as a target of inquiry in psychiatry, leading to a framework for care that is not fully responsive to the needs of patients. Section 2 provided a history of the evolution of the DSM's twin commitments. Section 3 examined the features of the current scientific framework for mental disorders, and Section 4 illustrated that the neglect of the self is expressed in the form of twin failures: the description of mental disorders in terms of behaviors isolated from the integrated complexity of the self who encounters them, and the underappreciation of the ability of patients' self-reports detailing the encounter with mental disorder to help develop scientific research on clinical interventions. The twin failures have been costly, both for psychiatry's clinical purposes and for patients' engagement and responses to their mental disorders. I turn to these costs in the next chapter.

Notes

1 I make a distinction between intervention and treatment. Intervention is a general category that delineates interactions between medical professionals and patients in which medical professionals prescribe measures that promote the health of patients. Treatment directly targets a patient's existing health problem (Steel and Tekin 2021). For example, vaccinations are examples of interventions while the prescription of antibiotics for tooth infection is an example of treatment. When I think of "interventions" in the context of psychiatry I am thus thinking about general measures to improve mental health or prevent mental disorder, while "treatments" are primarily about treating existing mental disorders.

2 There is disagreement amongst philosophers of psychiatry on whether Hempel's speech at the APA meeting genuinely influenced the changes in the diagnostic system. While some philosophers argue Hempel's operationalism was influential, others deny this historical argument (Cooper and Blashfield 2018; Tabb 2015; Tekin 2018). While it is beyond the scope of this book to take sides on this controversy, I believe that Hempel's talk, along with the larger conversations at the time about what it means for an area of inquiry to be scientific, as well as the enthusiasm about the medical model, created a perfect storm in which the DSM revisions were made.

3 There was wider reception of this idea in philosophical scholarship. For example, some philosophers argued the DSM was facing a crisis of public trust, and the inclusion of patients and individuals with a disability in the revision process would address the issue (Bueter 2018).

References

American Psychiatric Association. 1952. *Diagnostic and Statistical Manual of Mental Disorders*. 1st ed. Washington, DC: American Psychiatric Association.

American Psychiatric Association. 1968. *Diagnostic and Statistical Manual of Mental Disorders*. 1st ed. Washington, DC: American Psychiatric Association.

American Psychiatric Association. 1980. *Diagnostic and Statistical Manual of Mental Disorders*. 3rd ed. Washington, DC: American Psychiatric Association.

American Psychiatric Association. 1994. *Diagnostic and Statistical Manual of Mental Disorders*. 4th ed. Washington, DC: American Psychiatric Association.

American Psychiatric Association. 2000. *Diagnostic and Statistical Manual of Mental Disorders*. 4th ed. Text Revision. Washington, DC: American Psychiatric Association.

American Psychiatric Association. 2013. *Diagnostic and Statistical Manual of Mental Disorders*. 5th ed. Washington, DC: American Psychiatric Association.

Beck, Aaron T. 1962. Reliability of Psychiatric Diagnoses: 1. A Critique of Systematic Studies. *American Journal of Psychiatry* 119(3), 210–216. doi:10.1176/ajp.119.3.210.

Bluhm, Robyn. 2017. Evidence-Based Medicine, Biological Psychiatry, and the Role of Science in Medicine. In *Extraordinary Science and Psychiatry: Responses to the Crisis in Mental Health Research*, edited by J. Poland and Ş. Tekin, pp.37–57. Cambridge, MA: MIT Press.

Bridgman, P.W. 1938. Operational Analysis. *Philosophy of Science* 5(2), 114–131. doi:10.1086/286496.

Bueter, Anke. 2018. Public Epistemic Trustworthiness and the Integration of Patients in Psychiatric Classification. *Synthese* 198 (Suppl 19), 4711–4729. doi:10.1007/s11229-018-01913-z.

Chang, Hasok. 2019. Operationalism. In *Stanford Encyclopedia of Philosophy*. https://plato.stanford.edu/Entries/operationalism.

Cohen, Bruce J. 2003. *Theory and Practice of Psychiatry*. Oxford: Oxford University Press.

Cooper, John E., Robert E. Kendall, Barry J. Gurland, Norman Sartorius, and Tibor Farkas. 1969. Cross-National Study of the Diagnosis of the Mental Disorders: Some Results from the First Comparative Investigation. *American Journal of Psychiatry* 125(105), 21–29.

Cooper, Rachel and Roger Blashfield. 2018. The Myth of Hempel and the DSM-III. *Studies in History and Philosophy of Biological and Biomedical Sciences* 70, 10–19.

Cooper, R. and R. K. Blashfield. 2016. Re-Evaluating DSM-I. *Psychological Medicine* 46(3), 449–456. doi:10.1017/S0033291715002093.

Cuthbert, Bruce N. 2014. The RDoC Framework: Facilitating Transition from ICD/ DSM to Dimensional Approaches That Integrate Neuroscience and Psychopathology. *World Psychiatry* 13(1), 28–35. doi:10.1002/wps.20087.

Feighner, J.P., E. Robins, S.B. Guze, R.A. Woodruff, G. Winokur, and R. Munoz. 1972. Diagnostic Criteria for Use in Psychiatric Research. *Archives of General Psychiatry* 26(1), 57–63.

First, Michael B. 2010. Paradigm Shifts and the Development of the Diagnostic and Statistical Manual of Mental Disorders: Past Experiences and Future Aspirations. *The Canadian Journal of Psychiatry* 55(11), 692–700.

First, Michael B., Harold Alan Pincus, John B. Levine, Janet B.W. Williams, Bedirhan Ustun, and Roger Peele. 2004. Clinical Utility as a Criterion for Revising Psychiatric Diagnoses. *American Journal of Psychiatry* 161, 946–954.

Flanagan, Elizabeth H., Larry Davidson, and John S. Strauss. 2010. The Need for Patient-Subjective Data in the DSM and the ICD. *Psychiatry* 73(4), 297–307. doi:10.1521/psyc.2010.73.4.297.

Frank, Arthur W. 2005. *The Wounded Storyteller: Body, Illness & Ethics*. Chicago, IL: University of Chicago Press.

Freud, S. 1896. *History and the Aetiology of the Neuroses*. Redditch: Reads Books Limited, 2014.

Freud, S. 1917. Mourning and Melancholia. In *The Standard Edition of the Complete Psychological Works of Sigmund Freud*, edited by J. Strachey, pp. 243–258. London: Hogarth Press, 1957.

Goidsenhoven, Van Leni and Anneleen Masschelein. 2018. Donna Williams's 'Triumph': Looking for 'the Place in the Middle' at Jessica Kingsley Publishers. *Life Writing* 15(2), 171–193.

Graham, George and Owen Flanagan. 2013. Psychiatry and the Brain. Oxford University Blog. https://blog.oup.com/2013/08/psychiatry-brain-dsm-5-rdoc.

Grinker, Roy Richard. 2010. The Five Lives of the Psychiatry Manual. *Nature 468*, 168–170.

Grob, N. 1991. Origins of DSM-I: A Study in Appearance and Reality. *American Journal of Psychiatry* 148(4), 421–431.

Grünbaum, Adolf. 1984. *The Foundations of Psychoanalysis: A Philosophical Critique*: Berkeley, CA: University of California Press.

Guze, Samuel. 1978. Nature of Psychiatric Illness: Why Psychiatry Is a Branch of Medicine. *Comprehensive Psychiatry* 19(4), 295–307.

Guze, Samuel. 1992. *Why Psychiatry Is a Branch of Medicine*. Oxford: Oxford University Press.

Hempel, Carl. 1961. Introduction to Problems of Taxonomy. In *Field Studies in the Mental Disorders*, edited by J. Zubin, pp. 3–22. New York: Grune and Stratton, 1991.

Hoffman, Ginger and Peter Zachar. 2017. RDoC's Metaphysical Assumptions: Problems and Promises. In *Extraordinary Science and Psychiatry: Responses to the Crisis in Mental Health Research*, edited by J. Poland and Ş. Tekin, pp. 59–86. Cambridge, MA: MIT Press.

Horwitz, Allan V. 2015a. DSM-I and DSM-II. In *The Encyclopedia of Clinical Psychology*, edited by Robin L. Cautin and Scott O. Lilienfeld. Hoboken, NJ: Wiley-Blackwell.

Horwitz, Allan V. 2015b. How Did Everyone Get Diagnosed with Major Depressive Disorder?. *Perspectives in Biology and Medicine* 58 (1), 105–119. doi:10.1353/pbm.2015.0005.

Houts, Arthur C. 2000. Fifty Years of Psychiatric Nomenclature: Reflections on the 1943 War Department Technical Bulletin, Medical 203. *Journal of Clinical Psychology* 56(7), 935–967.

Hyman, Steven E. 2012. Revolution Stalled. *Science Translational Medicine* 4(155), 1–5.

Insel, Thomas. 2013. Transforming Diagnoses. *The National Institute of Mental Health Director's Blog* (blog). https://psychrights.org/2013/130429NIMHTransformingDiagnosis.htm.

Insel, Thomas. 2015. The Anatomy of NIMH Funding. *National Institute of Mental Health* (blog).

Insel, Thomas. 2022. *Healing: Our Path from Mental Illness to Mental Health*. Penguin Press.

Insel, T.R. and J.A. Lieberman. 2013. DSM-5 and RDoC: Shared Interests. *The National Institute of Mental Health* (blog). www.nimh.nih.gov/news/science-news/2013/dsm-5-and-rdoc-shared-interests.

Katz, Martin M., Jonathan O. Cole, and Walter E. Barton. 1968. *The Role and Methodology of Classification in Psychiatry and Psychopathology: Proceedings*. Washington, DC: U.S. Government Printing Office.

Kendler, Kenneth S., Rodrigo A. Muñoz, and George Murphy. 2010. The Development of the Feighner Criteria: A Historical Perspective. *The American Journal of Psychiatry* 167(2), 134–142. doi:10.1176/appi.ajp.2009.09081155.

Kuroki, Toshihide, M. Ishitobi, Y. Kamio, G. Sugihara, T. Murai, K. Motomura, K. Ogasawara, H. Kimura, B. Aleksic, N. Ozaki, T. Nakao, K. Yamada, K. Yoshiuchi, N. Kiriike, T. Ishikawa, C. Kubo, C. Matsunaga, H. Miyata, T. Asada, and S. Kanba. 2016. Current Viewpoints on DSM-5 in Japan. *Psychiatry and Clinical Neurosciences* 70, 371–393.

Murphy, Dominic. 2011. Conceptual Foundations of Biological Psychiatry. In *Philosophy of Medicine*, edited by Fred Gifford, pp. 425–451. Amsterdam: North-Holland.

National Institute of Mental Health. 2024. Important Events in NIMH History. www.nih.gov/about-nih/what-we-do/nih-almanac/national-institute-mental-health-nimh.

Popper, Karl R. 1959. *The Logic of Scientific Discovery*. New York: Basic Books.

Regier, Daniel A., Emily A. Kuhl, David J. Kupfer, and James P. McNulty. 2010. Patient Involvement in the Development of DSM-V. *Psychiatry: Interpersonal and Biological Processes* 73(4), 308–310.

Robins, Eli and Samuel B.Guze. 1970. Establishment of Diagnostic Validity in Psychiatric Illness: Its Application to Schizophrenia. *American Journal of Psychiatry* 126(7), 983–987.

Sadler, John Z. 2005. *Values and Psychiatric Diagnosis*. Oxford: Oxford University Press.

Sadler, John Z. and Bill Fulford. 2004. Should Patients and Their Families Contribute to the DSM-V Process?. *Psychiatric Services* 55(2), 113–204. doi:10.1176/appi. ps.55.2.133.

Sadler, J.Z., Osborne P. Wiggins, and Michael Alan Schwartz (Eds). 1994. Philosophical Perspectives on Psychiatric Classification. In *Philosophical Perspectives on Psychiatric Classification*, 315–331. Baltimore, MD: Johns Hopkins University Press.

Saks, Elyn R. 2007. *The Center Cannot Hold: My Journey Through Madness*. New York: Hachette Books.

Schechtman, Marya. 1997. *The Constitution of Selves*. Ithaca, NY: Cornell University Press.

Schwartz, Michael Alan and Osborne P. Wiggins. 1987a. Diagnosis and Ideal Types: A Contribution to Psychiatric Classification. *Comprehensive Psychiatry* 28(4), 277–291. doi:10.1016/0010-440X(87)90064-2.

Schwartz, Michael Alan, and Osborne P. Wiggins. 1987b. Typifications: The First Step for Clinical Diagnosis in Psychiatry. *The Journal of Nervous and Mental Disease* 175(2), 65–77. doi:10.1097/00005053-198702000-00001.

Slater, E. and M. Roth. 1969. *In Clinical Psychiatry*, edited by W. Mayer-Gross, E. Slater, and M. Roth, 3rd ed., pp. 272–287. London: Baillière, Tindall & Cassell.

Sokal, Robert R. 1974. Classification: Purposes, Principles, Progress, Prospects: Clustering and Other New Techniques Have Changed Classificatory Principles and Practice in Many Sciences. *Science* 185(4157), 1115–1123.

Solomon, Miriam. 2015. *Making Medical Knowledge*. Oxford: Oxford University Press.

Steel, Daniel and Şerife Tekin. 2021. Can Treatment for Substance Use Disorder Prescribe the Same Substance as That Used? The Case of Injectable Opioid Agonist Treatment. *Kennedy Institute of Ethics Journal* 31(3), 271–301.

Stein, Dan J. and Katharine A. Phillips. 2013. Patient Advocacy and DSM-5. *BMC Medicine* 11(133). doi:10.1186/1741-7015-11-133.

Suzuki, Yuriko et al. 2010. Comparison of Psychiatrists' Views on Classification of Mental Disorders in Four East Asian Countries/Area. *Asian Journal of Psychiatry* 3(1), 20–25.

Tabb, Kathryn. 2015. Psychiatric Progress and the Assumption of Diagnostic Discrimination. *Philosophy of Science* 82(5), 1047–1058. doi:10.1086/683439.

U.S. Department of Health and Human Services. 2024. *Fiscal Year 2025: Budget in Brief*. Washington, DC: U.S. Department of Health and Human Services. www. hhs.gov/sites/default/files/fy-2025-budget-in-brief.pdf.

Vaidyanathan, Uma. 2016. Facts and Myths about RDoC. Association for the Advancement of Philosophy and Psychiatry Annual Meeting, Atlanta, GA.

Watters, Ethan. 2010. *Crazy Like Us: The Globalization of the American Psyche*. New York: Free Press.

Chapter 3

Epistemic and ethical costs of neglecting the self in psychiatry

3.1 Introduction

This chapter builds on the arguments developed in the previous chapter and examines the implications of psychiatry's twin failures: first, describing mental disorders in terms of behaviors isolated from the integrated complexity of the self who encounters them, and second, not appreciating the ability of self-reports detailing the individual encounter with mental disorder to develop scientific research on clinical interventions. I argue these twin failures generate epistemic and ethical costs that make it difficult for individuals with mental disorder to flourish. Treatment plans guided by the DSM framework fall short of being resourceful in guiding the development of effective interventions for patients, and patients' self-narratives that are shaped by the DSM framework sometimes constrain their responses to their experiences.

The first part of the chapter explores the mechanisms through which the scientific frameworks in psychiatry shape the treatments patients receive and the way they think about their mental disorder, looking specifically at the mechanisms of the DSM's institutional and cultural power in clinical and personal contexts. The second part of the chapter outlines the epistemic and ethical costs of the twin failures for "flourishing," broadly defined as the development of subjects' psychological and social skills in interpreting and judging their relationships with themselves and others in the face of the circumstances in which they are placed, the demands of the world, and the challenges they are subject to therein. The acquisition of psychological and social skills that promote agency, i.e., individuals' capacity to act in the world as subjects, and autonomy, i.e., their ability to make informed and uncoerced decisions related to the states of affairs in their life, is closely connected to flourishing and enables individuals to live a responsible and fulfilling life.

DOI: 10.4324/9781003055556-5

3.2 Science to healthcare management: DSM's institutional power

The DSM is the most powerful document in contemporary psychiatry. As the introductions to the DSM-III, DSM-IV, and DSM-5 clearly indicate, the DSM is designed to be used for a variety of purposes and thus shapes numerous mental healthcare practices, research, education, and public thinking about mental disorders. Consider how the creators define these goals in the DSM-IV:

> Our highest priority has been to provide a helpful guide to clinical practice. We hoped to make DSM-IV practical and useful for clinicians by striving for brevity of criteria sets, clarity of language, and explicit statements of the constructs embodied in the diagnostic criteria. An additional goal was to facilitate research and improve communication among clinicians and researchers. We were also mindful of the use of DSM-IV for improving the collection of clinical information and as an educational tool for teaching psychopathology. An official nomenclature must be applicable in a wide diversity of contexts. DSM-IV is used by clinicians and researchers of many different orientations (e.g., biological, psychodynamic, cognitive, behavioral, interpersonal, family/systems). It is used by psychiatrists, other physicians, psychologists, social workers, nurses, occupational and rehabilitation therapists, counsellors, and other health and mental health professionals. DSM-IV must be usable across settings—inpatient, outpatient, partial hospital, consultation liaison, clinic, private practice, and primary care, and with community populations. It is also a necessary tool for collecting and communicating accurate public statistics. Fortunately, all these many uses are compatible with one another.
>
> (American Psychiatric Association 1994, xv)

The DSM-5 makes similar points but places more emphasis on concepts such as objectivity to underline its scientific commitment:

> The American Psychiatric Association's Diagnostic and Statistical Manual of Mental Disorders (DSM) is a classification of mental disorders with associated criteria designed to facilitate more reliable diagnoses of these disorders. With successive editions over the past 60 years, it has become a standard reference for clinical practice in the mental health field. Since a complete description of underlying pathological processes is not possible for mental disorders, it is important to emphasize that the current diagnostic criteria are the best available description of how mental disorders are expressed and can be recognized by trained clinicians. DSM is intended to serve as a practical,

functional, and flexible guide for organizing information that can aid in the accurate diagnosis and treatment of mental disorders. It is a tool for clinicians, an essential educational resource for students and practitioners, and a reference for researchers in the field. Although this edition of DSM was designed first and foremost to be a useful guide to clinical practice, as an official nomenclature it must be applicable in a wide diversity of contexts. DSM has been used by clinicians and researchers from different orientations (biological, psychodynamic, cognitive, behavioral, inter-personal, family/systems), all of whom strive for a common language to communicate the essential characteristics of mental disorders presented by their patients. The information is of value to all professionals asso-ciated with various aspects of mental health care, including psychiatrists, other physicians, psychologists, social workers, nurses, counselors, for-ensic and legal specialists, occupational and rehabilitation therapists, and other mental health professionals. The criteria are concise and explicit and intended to facilitate an objective assessment of symptom presenta-tions in a variety of clinical settings—inpatient, outpatient, partial hos-pital, consultation-liaison, clinical, private practice, and primary care—as well in general community epidemiological studies of mental disorders. DSM-5 is also a tool for collecting and communicating accurate public health statistics on mental disorder morbidity and mortality rates. Finally, the criteria and corresponding text serve as a textbook for stu-dents early in their profession who need a structured way to understand and diagnose mental disorders as well as for seasoned professionals encountering rare disorders for the first time. Fortunately, all of these uses are mutually compatible.

(American Psychiatric Association 2013, xli)

Thus, the DSM is designed to accomplish a plethora of pragmatic tasks across a variety of scientific and clinical settings: establishing clear and explicit criteria for mental disorders to assist clinical practice, facilitating research on mental disorders; improving communication among research-ers and healthcare practitioners, collecting clinical information over time, and creating an educational tool to teach psychopathology. It is intended to be used by scholars and practitioners, including clinicians and researchers in both inpatient and outpatient settings with different theore-tical orientations, such as psychiatrists, psychologists, social workers, nurses, therapists, and counsellors.

These myriad venues take the DSM beyond its clinical context, despite cautionary statements emphasizing the manual's intended use for clinical purposes. The DSM is clear: the diagnostic categories, criteria, and textual descriptions are meant to be employed by those with appropriate clinical training and experience in diagnosis and should not be applied by untrained persons (American Psychiatric Association 1994, xxiii). However, in practice, because it governs all aspects of mental health education, research, and care, the DSM carries a lot of institutional power and has influence beyond the clinic, thus magnifying both its benefits and its costs. Most notably, in the current healthcare system, a DSM diagnosis is required for insurance purposes: patients cannot get their healthcare expenses covered without a DSM diagnosis, and clinicians cannot be reimbursed unless they provide a DSM diagnosis for the patient. Even with an official diagnosis, the insurance coverage for mental health needs is suboptimal, encouraging patients and their families to seek knowledge and support from sources other than medical professionals, such as websites, blogs, movies, and even social media (e.g., Instagram reels, TikTok videos). As will be discussed, the cultural influence of the DSM on these various information channels magnifies the impact of the twin failures on patients.

In fact, the DSM's above-cited conviction that these different tasks are "not incompatible with each other" is false. First, the effort to make the DSM more scientific, with a focus on objective and easily measurable metrics such as observable behavior in lieu of the individual's historical and social context in which those behaviors emerge, means the DSM may not the best manual to guide clinicians in providing actual care for individuals. Knowing about an individual's history and social relationships might be relevant to how clinicians engage with the patient, as well as the kind of mental healthcare they provide. Second, when it is used as a guide by individuals to make sense of their mental disorder experience, it may constrain their resources for flourishing. The easily measurable metrics such as behavior might lead patients to be overconcerned about their symptoms and unable to situate those symptoms in the wider net of their mental states and lives. We need a bridge between the DSM framework and patients with a mental disorder to promote patients' flourishing. More precisely, we need to provide clinicians and patients with cognitive and practical tools to engage with mental disorders so that patients can flourish.

3.3 Science to TikTok: DSM's cultural power

Beyond the clinical context, the DSM has become the standard framework for understanding and engaging with mental disorders more generally. Its cultural impact can be examined through the lens of what philosopher Ian Hacking calls the "looping effects" of scientific classifications (Hacking 1986, 1995a). He uses this phenomenon to discuss what he calls "making up people," i.e., the ways scientific classifications made by human sciences may bring a new kind of person into being (e.g., Hacking 1986, 1995a, 1995b, 1999, 2004, 2007a, 2007b). Looping effects have two arcs: the first comprises the influence of scientific classifications on those so classified; the second comprises the ways some classified individuals respond to and modify the systems of classification. Scientific classifications alter the way individuals think about themselves and their behavior; this, in turn, destabilizes the initial classification, in that the category becomes no longer applicable to an individual's experiences and forces scientists to redefine and change their classifications. Some people with mental disorders (e.g., multiple personality and schizophrenia) are subject to the looping effects of psychiatric classifications, but looping effects are not restricted to the domain of mental disorders. Hacking also mentions female refugees, pregnant teenagers, child abusers, the obese, and the genius (see e.g., Hacking 1986, 1995a, 1995b, 2007a, 2007b; Tekin 2014a).

Let's break down the process whereby scientific classifications offered by the human sciences induce changes in the subjects they study. The goal of these sciences is to acquire systematic, general, and accurate knowledge about puzzling and idiosyncratic phenomena pertaining to human beings in "industrialized bureaucracies"—for example, suicide, child abuse, multiple personality, obesity, and refugee status. Human sciences seek to attain "generalizations sufficiently strong that they seem like laws about people, their actions, or their sentiments" so that helpful interventions can be made (Hacking 1995a, 352). However, unlike the objects of inquiry in natural sciences, the subjects of human sciences—i.e., human kinds—respond to how they are classified. Hacking distinguishes between human and natural kinds by noting that human kinds are subject to looping effects, owing to the "self-awareness" of at least some of those classified:

> Responses of people to attempts to be understood or altered are different from the responses of things. This trite fact is at the core of one difference between the natural and human sciences, and it works at the level of kinds. There is a looping or feedback effect involving the introduction to classifications of people. New sorting and theorizing induces changes in self-conception and in behaviour of the people classified. Those changes demand revisions of the classifications and theories, the causal connections, and the expectations. Kinds are modified, revised classifications are formed, and the classified change again, loop upon a loop.
>
> (Hacking 1995a, 370)

Hacking's best-known example of looping effects is multiple personality disorder, previously an official diagnosis in the DSM but removed in the DSM-IV, owing largely to worries about its scientific credibility, and replaced by dissociative identity disorder. Multiple personality, broadly stated, refers to experiences of individuals who involuntarily display multiple personalities at different times and in different contexts. These personalities, at times featuring opposite properties, seem to appear and disappear on their own, without the individual's control; patients often report not remembering what their "alter" personality does. The diagnosis of multiple personality disorder is a medically, socially, and culturally puzzling challenge to the idea that each individual body possesses one mind/personality. Hacking calls it a "microcosm of thinking-and-talking about making-up people" and uses it to show how "the sciences of the soul," in their attempts to make the soul an object of scientific query, make up people (1986, 1995a, 1995b).

Hacking observes that the symptoms characterizing multiple personality disorder changed as knowledge of the illness entered popular culture under the combined influence of curious psychiatrists, television show producers, and patient alliances. As Hacking sees it, those diagnosed with multiple personality started displaying different symptoms as they learned more about the illness and its manifestations in different individuals through popular culture. For example, in the early days, individuals displayed one or two alternate personalities, but as the phenomenon became popular, individuals displayed numerous personalities and at times animal personalities (Hacking 1995b). In other words, the behaviors individuals displayed fit the popular descriptions of this condition. The changes in the behaviors they displayed, in turn, altered the classification of multiple personality.

The looping effects related to multiple personality disorder took the following shape:

Step 1: Psychiatry (as a human science) acquires systematic knowledge (K1) about human subjects (S1) who exhibit alternating personalities that are amnesic to one another. K1 picks out the perceived law-like regularities in S1 (e.g., alternating personalities).

Step 2: On the basis of K1, psychiatry forms classifications (CL1) of S1, labeling S1 "persons with multiple personality."

Step 3: At least some individuals with multiple personality (S1a) become aware of their categories, as K1 is disseminated in popular culture through the combined impact of psychiatrists, television show producers, alliances of S1a, and so on (Hacking 1999, 106). Informed by K1, S1a change their behavior (b) and self-concepts (c).

Step 4: The awareness of being classified, the changes in the behavior, and the changes in the self-concepts of those classified (S1a) amount to changes in the perceived regularities about these people. S1a start to feature new symptoms not found in S1, for example, exhibiting animal personalities.

Step 5: Changes in the perceived regularities of S1a lead to changes in K1 about their CL1, because S1a no longer fit the criteria for CL1.

Summary: The scientific classifications and the individuals so classified influence and change each other through the interactive and iterative process of looping effects. Classification of some individuals as "people with multiple personality" results in the creation of new knowledge (K1a), new classifications (CL1a), and new kinds of people (S1a).

In his later work, Hacking expanded the nexus of looping effects to include "experts" who engage in scientific research, "institutions" where interactions occur between experts and classified individuals, and the "knowledge" generated in this process. Each node in this nexus exerts an influence on the other nodes. Experts influence the subjects they study or treat; similarly, the institutions in which these exchanges occur influence the subjects' self-concepts and behavior. All these influences shape the knowledge generation process in human sciences. Thus, the causal net of looping effects, according to this new framework, is much wider than originally thought (Tekin 2014a).

The concept of looping effects provides a helpful lens through which to understand how the DSM, as a cultural force, shapes the ways society and its institutions understand and respond to mental disorders. Through the mechanism of looping effects, the DSM is instrumental in forming the DSM culture, i.e., the interactive cultural context in which DSM-oriented psychiatric knowledge is widely distributed to and accepted by the public (Tekin 2011). The elements of the DSM culture include not only the mental healthcare teams or researchers noted in the DSM's introduction, but also the institutions, patients, caregivers, and individuals impacted by mental disorders more generally. The list includes the following: people experiencing mental distress who are subject to DSM classifications and their caregivers; experts who conduct research on mental disorders in various capacities (e.g., researchers on the DSM task forces, psychiatrists who diagnose subjects and provide treatment plans, scientists who seek to discover the roots of mental disorders, and social workers who aid medication management); experts who are treating or training to treat patients (e.g., psychiatrists, family doctors, residents, and medical school students); and institutions that administer research and care (e.g., American Psychiatric Association, National Institute of Mental Health, pharmaceutical companies, insurance firms, and local clinics). These experts collectively generate knowledge about mental disorders. This knowledge guides and is guided by the DSM schema; it is incorporated into the DSM classifications, clinical research experiments, and the development of treatment methods, such as psychotropic drugs. In this way, the DSM's approach to mental disorders is formed, used, and disseminated in a wider DSM culture.

These dynamic interactions take the DSM's twin failures, i.e., its hyponarrativity, through its focus on a set of behaviors isolated from the integrated complexity of the self who encounters a mental disorder and its underappreciation of patients' perspectives, beyond the clinical context in which the DSM is intended to be used. For example, an increasing number of self-help media take the DSM criteria as definitive descriptions of mental disorders (even though the DSM is clear that these are provisional categories as research on mental disorders continues) and use them to give advice. A quick search on TikTok reveals numerous videos recorded by teenagers who either diagnose themselves with a mental disorder, going through the DSM criteria for certain conditions on-screen, or telling others how to diagnose themselves. It is far from clear whether these teenagers genuinely encounter experiences that can be diagnosed by clinicians, such as bipolar disorder or posttraumatic stress disorder (PTSD), or whether they are simply bored or struggling with who they are and who they want to become and seeking some kind of external validation by making themselves more interesting or attention-worthy. What cannot be contested is that they need guidance and support: either genuine clinical support if they have bipolar disorder or PTSD, or personal and social support if they are using these self-narratives to discover who they are, or a combination of both. Leaving their care to the DSM terminology or framework is doing them an injustice; we need to create pathways through which they can understand their experiences and respond to them in a way that will enable flourishing. I return to this issue in Chapter 5, when I discuss how the Multitudinous Self Model (*MuSe*) can provide resources to clinicians and patients.

Thus, as philosopher Jeffrey Poland suggests, the DSM ends up informing "how an important domain of human suffering, disability, and deviance is observed, understood, and engaged" by a broader public (Poland 2001). Consequently, as I go on to show, the individuals diagnosed as having mental disorders are subject to the epistemic and ethical costs generated by psychiatry's twin failures. Owing to the DSM's hyponarrativity, individuals with mental disorders are sometimes unable to situate their experiences in the larger complexity of their selfhood, as hyponarrative descriptions come to dominate their narratives about their mental disorder experiences and constrain their flourishing. Similarly, because the DSM's knowledge generation process excludes patients' expertise in understanding and managing mental disorders, the institutional contexts in which they are cared for result in situations where their autonomy and agency are undermined. Hyponarrative approaches to mental disorders pervade medical education and clinical training, and clinicians are not trained about the full complexity of the selfhood and the complex and thick aspects of a life with various distresses. In addition, because the first-person expertise of patients is not made part of psychiatric knowledge, clinicians are not adequately aware of what works and what does not work in clinical contexts. In light of these failures, clinicians may not be willing to trust patients' self-reports of their experiences simply because what they are pointing out is not in the official nomenclature of DSM-generated psychiatric knowledge; this sometimes leads them to ignore patients' reports, preventing them from truly addressing their concerns.

3.4 Epistemic and ethical costs of psychiatry's twin failures for flourishing

Psychiatry's twin failures have epistemic and ethical costs for patients' flourishing by shaping clinical interventions through what I call the "therapeutic" impact of psychiatric diagnoses and by shaping patients' own understanding of their mental disorders through what I call the "reflective" impact (Tekin 2014b).

First, let's consider the therapeutic impact. As I have explained, the fundamental goal of scientific research in psychiatry is to develop effective clinical interventions, but this goal is not met because the lack of self-related phenomena in the scientific framework results in an incomplete picture of mental disorders in the clinic. The DSM's criteria for diagnosing mental disorders leave out important features of the individual that can and do contribute to their mental disorder onset, ranging from biological constitution and personal history to identity-constituting dimensions, such as race, gender, and socioeconomic status, not to mention the social context in which they are embedded. The DSM framework, widely used in medical education and clinical training programs, does not provide clinicians with the tools they need to engage with the self-related complexities of their patients' encounter with mental disorders. In addition, because the patients themselves are not officially part of the development process of the DSM, their insights into their mental disorders and their care are not made part of psychiatric knowledge. Accordingly, clinicians do not learn how the identity-constituting properties of the self intersect with the properties of mental distresses and disorders. Knowing about the person's interests, past, family dynamics, relationship status, and so on, at least minimally, opens a window into what the patient may be experiencing and may suggest resources for the clinician to connect with the patient and partner with them on the path to recovery.

However, there are no guidelines for the clinician to engage the patient in this way. Instead, clinical interactions often focus on going over the standard criteria for a mental disorder diagnosis by asking generic questions. In addition, as the DSM is used for teaching purposes in medical schools and residency programs, its framework shapes what professionals learn. Medical students and psychiatry residents are not likely to receive special training in engaging with the complexity and identity-constituting features of the patient's self, as the symptom-management approach promoted by the DSM lends itself to a medication-based treatment strategy and does not provide guidelines for other forms of treatment. As anthropologist Tanya Luhrmann clearly demonstrates in *Of Two Minds: An Anthropologist Looks at American Psychiatry,* most residency programs in psychiatry focus on neuroscience, psychopharmacology, and medication management. Teaching medical students how to interact with patients or how to offer psychotherapy and other forms of treatments takes a back seat (Luhrmann 2001). Not much has changed since Luhrmann's observations at the turn of the century. A quick survey of medical school and psychiatric residency curricula in the leading institutions in the United States (e.g., Johns Hopkins University, Columbia University, New York University, and University of Pennsylvania) shows that as of early 2025, students are not taught about the self, cultural diversity, and cognition in a systematic way. While many courses cover neuroscience, and some cover psychodynamic theory, there is no coverage of research in cognitive science on the nature of the self or human cognition. The tools to engage with patients in the clinic or guides on to how to diagnose, what to diagnose, when to diagnose are also sporadic. Some institutions require students to take "motivational interviewing" training, a technique that medical professionals use to help people recognize their problems and motivate them to do something about them, but this is not standard practice. In addition, it is questionable whether motivational interviewing really engages with the features of the self in a systematic basis. Thus, DSM's twin failures result in an impoverished therapeutic impact because clinicians are not provided with the education and tools that they need to engage with the complexity of the self they encounter in the clinic.

An impoverished representation of mental disorders, devoid of the complexity and richness of the self, can impede flourishing through the reflective impact of psychiatric diagnoses (Tekin 2014b). The authoritative nature of a psychiatric diagnosis, by virtue of being delivered by scientifically and clinically trained experts in a care institution, and the perceived plausibility of the explanations offered by the DSM, give DSM-based information the power to influence patients' self-reflections. In this sense, the DSM not only has a therapeutic impact on patients by way of organizing how their mental disorders are therapeutically addressed by clinicians; it also has a reflective impact on how these patients make sense of their lived experiences: how they understand their mental disorder diagnoses, their interpersonal relationships, and other important components of their lives, and most importantly, how they respond to these states of affairs in their self-narratives.

Patients' reflections on themselves shape their relationships and their lives in general and influence their responses to their mental distresses or disorders. "Self-narratives" are selective representations of the states of affairs in an individual's life, organized in a more or less sequential, coherent, and meaningful manner and expressed through language (Tekin 2011, 2014b). They serve as cognitive tools for making sense of things, including past experiences of mental disorder, trauma, or violence (Baylis 2011; Flanagan 1996; Jopling 2000; Lindemann Nelson 2001; Lumsden 2013; Tekin 2010, 2011, 2014b; Tekin and Mosko 2015). In addition to expressing individuals' conceptions of their experiences, self-narratives shape their responses to them, for better or for worse.

For instance, following a breakup, a young woman may reiterate the series of events leading to the breakup, reexamine the role played by each partner, identify potential reasons for the breakup, etc. Such self-narratives help her to get a grasp on what happened. These self-narratives, incomplete and selective by nature, have varying degrees of connection with the states of affairs that have actually occurred: they may be veridical or far removed from the reality. In this respect, they are plastic; they are influenced not only by the actual events, but also by the social, cultural, and scientific norms that evaluate them. After reading a book in a class about gender dynamics in relationships, the woman may create another version of the self-narrative about the relationship and the breakup. Creating a narrative that makes sense of it through an understanding of power relations many help her adjust and overcome negative experiences associated with the relationship, such as abuse, in a more resourceful way. Alternatively, she may make sense of the breakup by focusing on her own features and role in the relationship (as opposed to looking at the partner's behavior) and create a self-narrative that characterizes her as unworthy of a relationship. Such self-narratives may damage the woman's self-respect and self-regard, limiting possible responses to the breakup.

Social narratives, i.e., other people's narratives of the states of affairs in an individual's life, can be made part of self-narratives as well (Tekin 2011, 2013). Depending on their quality, they may help or hinder the individual's adjustment to the events in their lives, shaping their available cognitive and social resources (Jopling 2000). There are salient examples throughout human history of dominant groups shaping the narratives of certain under-represented groups, "damaging" their identity so that they cannot exercise their moral agency freely (Lindemann Nelson 2001). For example, if the abovementioned woman's self-narrative highlights the partner's insistence on her negative personality traits and posits these as the sole reason for the breakup, she may develop feelings of insecurity that hinder flourishing.

A DSM diagnosis shapes both self-narratives and social narratives. An encounter with a mental disorder is expressed as a form of orientational challenge: the raw experience of encountering a mental disorder on physical, social, and conceptual levels directly affects the way individuals orient themselves in the world. They might have trouble falling asleep or getting up in the morning or may struggle to stay focused at work. They may be reluctant to see their close friends and develop feelings of worthlessness or insecurity. A DSM diagnosis influences self-narratives about these orientational challenges (Tekin 2014b). For example, upon being diagnosed with major depressive disorder, the individual may redefine their past experiences based on the descriptive framework established by the diagnostic schema, reassess the psychological and historical facts of their life in light of the theory underlying the diagnosis, start to reevaluate certain past events as earlier symptoms of the mental disorder, and so on. After being diagnosed, they may make better sense of, say, their increasing sadness, significant weight loss, insomnia, and suicidal thoughts exacerbated by feelings of hopelessness and despair in early adulthood. This understanding may lead them to reassess a failure in their first job as an outcome of mental disorder, instead of, say, incompetence. The alteration in the subject's autobiographical narrative may generate changes in their future plans, hopes, desires, anticipations, expectations, and habits, as well as their relationships with others. They may, for instance, blame a failed relationship on their depression.

Consider the effect of being diagnosed with major depressive disorder on self-narrative in the following passage from Daphne Merkin's "A Journey through Darkness":

> I do know that by the age of 5 or 6, in my corduroy overalls, racing around in Keds, I had begun to be apprehensive about what lay in wait for me. I felt that events had not conspired in my favor, for many reasons, including the fact that in my family there were too many children and too little attention to go around. What attention there was came mostly from an abusive nanny who scared me into total compliance and a mercurial mother whose interest was often unkindly. By age 8, I was wholly unwilling to attend school, out of some combination of fear and separation anxiety. (It seems to me now, many years later, that I was expressing early on a chronic depressive's wish to stay home, on the inside, instead of taking on the outside, loomingly hostile world in the form of classmates and teachers.) By 10 I had been hospitalized because I cried all the time, although I don't know if the word "depression" was ever actually used.
>
> (Merkin 2009)

The diagnosis of major depressive disorder in adulthood helped Merkin make sense of the mental distress of her early childhood. It helped her reevaluate what happened then and thus functions as a form of explanation in her autobiographical narrative. In other words, the diagnosis of depression made her experiences palpable and understandable.

The DSM diagnosis also affects social narratives about the subject, allowing others to reconceptualize the individual's actions, temper, and personality traits using the explanatory paradigm offered by the diagnosis. Ruth White's 2008 narrative is a good illustration of this point. She reports that she received a diagnosis of attention deficit and hyperactivity disorder. A year later, following a rough period involving her mental health, she received a diagnosis of bipolar disorder. In addition to affecting White herself, the change in the diagnosis affected her friends:

> It was too difficult, too, for many of those same friends… to accept this new diagnosis. They questioned whether I was not simply stressed out from the many changes that had been going on in my life: a new job, a new city, my partner's move, and my new single-motherhood status. Ironically some of my friends thought that I was just being over-medicalized and overmedicated. That angered me. … For my friends to think that I was basically being emotionally lazy hurt me deeply. I knew that if I had called to say that I had cancer, the response would have been significantly different. I would have received empathy instead of being challenged on the validity of my diagnosis.
>
> (White 2008, 49)

White's points are telling. The change in her diagnosis made her friends question the perceived reality of her experience of the mental disorder. This, in turn, affected how White perceived her puzzled psychological states, her coping, her friendships, and her professional performance. Thus, the social narrative directly affected the self-narrative.

Used as a cognitive tool, a DSM-informed self-narrative can be used to make sense of otherwise unfathomable mental distress. On the one hand, a DSM diagnosis situates experience in an established classificatory system which can facilitate self-understanding by providing insight into the subject's condition and giving a direction to treatment and recovery. In this sense, the DSM diagnosis may have positive ramifications for the processes of recovery and may positively affect the subject's self-perception. On the other hand, given DSM's twin failures, a diagnosis may direct the subject to make sense of their distress divorced from other elements in their life that may be affecting their mental health and may guide them to frame their experience as an unchangeable phenomenon. This form of self-understanding may set limits on the subject's hopes of recovery and preclude flourishing. For example, instead of framing their experiences as sadness as a result of underappreciation at work, and searching for other work, the subject might think of their experiences as being depressed. Instead of trying to address the issue on a practical level, say, by talking to an employer or looking for another job, they may ignore the source of the problem and turn to medical treatments for depression (Tekin 2011, 2014b).

The following self-narrative by Stephanie Foo demonstrates the reflective impact of psychiatric diagnoses on self-narratives and their potential limitations:

> In the past week I've been scrolling through various mental illnesses on WebMD, searching for symptoms that sound familiar to find an answer. Now, near the end of my session with Samantha [the thera-pist] ... I gather up my courage to ask about my internet diagnosis. "Do you think I am bipolar?" Samantha actually laughs. "You are not bipolar. I am sure of it," she says. ... "Do you want to know your diagnosis?" ... I say, "Yes. Of course." Something in her jaw becomes determined, and her gaze is direct. "You have complex PTSD from your childhood, and it manifests as persistent depression and anxiety." ... The first thing I do after our Skype window closes is to bring up Google. I've never heard of complex PTSD. Surprisingly, there aren't that many results. I go from Wikipedia to a government page about C-PTSD as it relates to veterans. I read the list of symptoms. It is very long. And it is not so much a medical document as it is a biography of my life: The difficulty regulating my emotions. The tendency to over-share and trust the wrong people. The dismal self-loathing. The trouble I have maintaining relationships. The unhealthy relationship with my

abuser. The tendency to be aggressive but unable to tolerate aggression from others. It's all true. It's all me. The more I read. The more every aspect of my personhood is reduced to deep diagnostic flaws. I hadn't understood how far the disease had spread. How complete its takeover of my identity was. The things I want. The things I love. The way I speak. My passions, my fears, my zits, my eating habits, the amount of whiskey I drink, the way I listen, and the things I see. Everything—everything, all of it—is infected. My trauma is literally pumping through my blood, driving every decision in my brain.

(Foo 2022, xiii–xiv)

While a PTSD diagnosis gave a conceptual framework for Foo to think about her past experiences, I worry that she is "reducing" her entire personality to "diagnostic flaws," or is considering the things she wants, dreams of, and is passionate about in terms of trauma. It is unclear how thinking about her passions and dreams in terms of her mental disorder will give her resources to flourish. Setting her traumatic experiences within the broader richness of her life as the daughter of immigrants, successful podcast-maker, etc. might yield more resources to encounter challenges and respond to them.

Let's return to one of the examples in Chapter 1; in this passage, Elyn Saks explains how she situated her experiences within a DSM-based narrative:

I had discovered the DSM. ... I read it cover to cover. Knowledge had always been my salvation, but with my immersion into the DSM, I began to understand that there were some truths that were too difficult and frightening to know. ... And now, here it was, in writing: The Diagnosis. What did it mean? Schizophrenia is a brain disease which entails a profound loss of connection to reality. It is often accompanied with delusions, which are fixed yet false beliefs—such as you have killed thousands of people—and hallucinations, which are false sensory perceptions—such as you have just seen a man with a knife. Often speech and reason can become disorganized to the point of incoherence. The prognosis: I would largely lose the capacity to take care of myself. I wasn't expected to have a career, or even a job that might bring in a pay check. I wouldn't be able to form attachments, or keep friendships, or find someone to love me, or have a family of my own—in short I'd never have a life. ... I'd always been optimistic that when and if the mystery of me was solved, it could be fixed; now I was being told that whatever had gone wrong inside my head was permanent, and from all indications, unfixable. Repeatedly, I ran up against words like "debilitating," "baffling," "chronic," "catastrophic," "devastating" and "loss." For the rest of my life. The rest of my life. It felt more like a death sentence than a medical diagnosis.

(Saks 2007, 167–168)

Saks's self-narrative echoes the formal definition of schizophrenia found in the DSM and reflects the speculative and unverified knowledge about schizophrenia disseminated in the DSM culture. For instance, the DSM does not say schizophrenia is a brain disease, but the substantive literature on schizophrenia, including research articles, pharmaceutical studies, neuroscientific literature, not to mention popular literature, refers to it as such. Some terms, including "permanent," "debilitating," "catastrophic," are not found in the DSM. This particular self-narrative is constraining, as it accounts for Saks's experiences with hallucinations and delusions superficially, without engaging with how these states are lived out in different contexts of her life. For instance, it is relevant to the development of Saks's understanding of and response to her illness that she know the times she is more disposed to certain hallucinations, for example, the highly stressful examinations at Oxford, so that she can develop ways to deal with them. However, a symptom-oriented narrative does not engage with those factors.

The kind of self-narrative that disengages Saks' symptoms from her larger life context might shut down other, more integrated accounts of her experience with schizophrenia. In fact, Saks has a fulfilling life despite her illness, demonstrating her ability to create alternative, more integrated self-narratives in which she is not a collection of symptom clusters, but an individual person with a meaningful life. Saks writes in her memoir that she has flourished by replacing the above narratives with more resourceful ones where she engages with the meaning of her illness and its significance in her life. In other words, not relying on the DSM-based criteria has helped her.

In short, the elimination of the subjective dimensions of the patient's experiences, including interpersonal, developmental, socioeconomic, and environmental factors, and the assumption that the mental disorder is running its course at least somewhat independently of these other personal contingencies, might pose serious problems for the patient's grasp of their mental disorder if the diagnosis is used as a reflective tool. Hyponarrativity, if incorporated into the patient's self-reflection, will direct them to focus on symptoms, undermining the importance of their unique life and contributing to limitations in responding to mental disorders. In this respect, symptom-oriented thinking about mental disorders might lead individuals to emphasize their symptoms at the expense of undermining their personal identity and interpersonal relationships when thinking about their lived experience in the world.

Perhaps we can think about this phenomenon as patients' adopting a "medical stance" towards themselves. The term "medical stance" follows Daniel Dennett's (1971) concept of an "intentional stance," referring to the level of abstraction through which we view the behavior of an individual in terms of their mental states, such as beliefs and desires. Dennett suggests that to predict a person's behavior, we must first assume this person is a rational agent who acts according to their beliefs and desires (Dennett 1971).

Dennett's concept of an intentional stance is developed in the context of his work on folk psychology, which he believes provides a systematic "reason-giving explanation" for an agent's behavior. In making sense of the individual's behavior, we, as the folk, make certain assumptions about the agent, that their action is rational and reasonable in the circumstances, that they have certain beliefs and desires, and that their future action can be systematically predicted from the beliefs and desires so ascribed. By adopting the intentional stance, then, we might predict an agent's behavior based on our assumptions about their rationality and mental states.[1] When we use intentional stance to explain people's behavior, we are concerned with such things as belief, thinking, and intent. When we predict the cat will run away because it knows a stranger is coming and is afraid of them, we are taking an intentional stance. Another example would be when we predict Alice will leave the meeting at two pm and take a Lyft to the airport because she wants to arrive at the airport on time for her 5 pm flight. Thus, we can say that sometimes, DSM-led medical framework for mental disorders leads the individual to adopt a medical stance towards their experiences, preventing them from making sense of their experiences or reflecting on their challenges by using non-medical stances.

Note that the way the DSM-based knowledge shapes an individual's self-reflection is not entirely due to the top-down effect of psychiatric diagnoses on the individual. It is also due to the complex architecture of human cognition which shapes how human beings interpret, understand, and use the information they receive from the environment. This is precisely why it is important to study the self in thinking about mental disorders. I develop this more fully in Chapter 4, but for now, let me look at one feature of our cognition that makes possible the more or less resourceful ways of making sense of our experiences.

Traditionally, unbounded rationality was considered the norm of human cognitive processes involved in moral, social, and intellectual judgment, and rational decision-making was identified with logic. The self was considered an unbounded rational unity, immune to irrationalities, instabilities, and inconsistencies. An unboundedly rational person was assumed to be omniscient, with unlimited computational power, able to acquire complete knowledge from their environment and make unbiased and objective decisions about the states of affairs in their lives (Gigerenzer 2006). However, this picture leaves out the mental and environmental limitations of human cognition. Empirical research in cognitive and social psychology increasingly challenges traditional philosophical assumptions about the nature of our cognitive mechanisms, pointing to short-sighted reasoning strategies, biases, and opportunistic oversimplifications (Gilovich 1993; Kahneman et al. 1982; Wilson 2002). Studies have shown humans consistently make errors of judgment, that is, systematic deviations from rationality (e.g., Gilbert 2006).

To better understand why DSM-led psychiatric knowledge might constrain the individual epistemically, consider the subjective validation effect, also known as the Barnum effect. This cognitive bias is defined as the tendency of subjects to identify their personal features with broad or vague characterizations of their personality, even when such characterizations are not veridical (Dmitruk et al. 1973). A paradigmatic example is a subject's response to what is said about them in personality profiles, astrological projections, and the like. Even though the descriptions are vague and general enough to be applicable to a large number of people, some believe they are veridical reflections of who they are, and the features are unique to them (e. g., Dmitruk et al. 1973). The statements from personality profiles involve such observations as, "You have a great need for other people to like and admire you" (Jopling 2000, 40). Nothing is unique or specific to a particular subject, yet many believe this is a valid characterization of their unique personality. Subjects will also accept such broad and vague descriptions as accurate if the analysis is offered by an authoritative agent (Dickson and Kelly 1985). The influence of the DSM-led psychiatric knowledge that prioritizes symptoms at the expense of subjectivity in mood disorder descriptions might trigger a similar kind of cognitive bias in the patient. Because these descriptions are general, lack detail, and leave no room for particular contingencies, patients, when exposed to such information via various media of the DSM culture, might overidentify their experiences with the suggested symptoms, undermining other, more personal aspects of their lives. Some patients, upon being informed of the symptoms of mood disorders, might start making sense of their lived experience with a skewed focus on the symptoms. By attending to their symptoms and ignoring other essential components of their lives, such as personal identity and interpersonal relationships, they might attribute the sources of their interpersonal problems to their symptoms, not to other fundamental ingredients of their lives. In other words, cognitive bias, such as the Barnum effect, puts them at risk of over-attending to symptoms of illness at the expense of undermining personal identity and interpersonal relationships in self-narratives.

Another way of making sense of the DSM's influence on self-narratives is to use the concept of "value capture" developed by philosopher Thi Nguyen. According to Nguyen, while an individual's own values are rich and subtle, when they enter certain social environments, they take on board and internalize the value metrics promulgated by these environments. In Nguyen's words, they "internalize" these metrics (Nguyen 2024). His examples include being motivated by Fitbit's step counts, Twitter likes, citation rates, and so on. In value capture, individuals take a certain component of their autonomy and decision-making process and outsource it to a large-scale institution's value system that is developed for purposes of measurability and is aggregable. This cuts the individual off from their own values and articulations "in light of their own rich experience of the world," and they stop tailoring their values to their selves or goals (Nguyen 2024). The DSM framework serves as an institutional value capture system in that it dominates an individual's values, defining which kinds of behaviors are healthy or unhealthy. As the above self-narratives indicate, the influence of the DSM can sometimes lead individuals to evaluate themselves and their life experiences through the DSM's value capture, as opposed to their own rich value systems. For example, initially, Saks's life as an individual with schizophrenia did not look promising under the DSM's value capture: because she had schizophrenia, she was unlikely to hold a job or develop nurturing relationships. Her life experiences were described by words like "debilitating," "baffling," "chronic," "catastrophic," "devastating," and "loss." If she chose to adopt the DSM-style values, she might have ended up in a life that would not allow her flourish and be fulfilled. Instead of using the DSM's value capture, however, she designed her own life, finding a niche as a person with schizophrenia, creating a rich personal value system which helped her flourish.

Another example of the way the DSM's influence on self-narratives can inhibit flourishing is found in Terry Cheney's memoir of her bipolar disorder. She says she received various diagnoses, starting at the age of 16, including an eating disorder, depression, and bipolar disorder. She was hospitalized a few times, attempted suicide, and received electroconvulsive therapy (ECT). It took her a long time to receive "the most accurate diagnosis" of her puzzling mental health problems (Cheney 2009, 20). She suspected she might have bipolar disorder and consulted self-help books. After reading a self-help book on mood disorders and noticing that her puzzling mental states overlapped with the symptoms of bipolar disorder, she says she self-diagnosed:

> Something was wrong with me, I suspected; I just didn't have the name for it yet. I hated the world, I hated myself, and dying sounded just fine to me: all classic symptoms of depression. But—and it was a crucial but—I could still move. Not only *could* I move, I *had* to move. I was full of restless, undissipated energy that had no place to go, making me want to strike out and break something, preferably something that would crash and tinkle into a thousand satisfying tiny pieces.... It took me a few more hours, and several more books, but I finally found it: the solution to the mystery, the clinical term for what was wrong with me. Apparently, there's a strange state on the bipolar spectrum called a "mixed state," in which mania and depression meet and collide. In a mixed state, you have all the relentless, agitated drive of mania, but none of the euphoria. Instead you feel depression's misery and self-loathing. It's the most dangerous condition possible, the one in which the most suicides occur. No longer protected by depression's inertia, you now have the ability to act upon your despair. There it was, in

black and white: my absolution. I wasn't crazy. It wasn't depression, it wasn't even mania. It was a mixed state. I was entitled to feel horrible, it was a mixed state. I kept saying the term over and over to myself on the way back to the hotel, to make it real.

(Cheney 2009, 184–185)

Cheney accepted what she thought was a plausible explanation for her experiences. This diagnosis was later confirmed by her psychiatrist.

The diagnosis and the terminology used in the DSM set the tone of Cheney's writing; within this conceptual framework, she interprets and shares her encounter with bipolar disorder. In the section where she gives the reasons for writing her memoir, she suggests:

That's why I've chosen to tell my life story episodically, rather than in any chronological order. It is truer to the way I think. When I look back, I rarely remember events in terms of date or sequence. Rather, I remember what emotional state I was in. Manic? Depressed? Suicidal? Euphoric? Life for me is defined not by time, but by mood.

(Cheney 2009, 1)

This paragraph, disclosing her retrospective reasoning about her mood disorder, has traces of a DSM-led framework. It hints at hyponarrativity and the elimination of the consideration of complex cognitive architecture in thinking about her condition; she reveals little about her psychological distress as it relates to the particular aspects of her life, such as her identity and her interpersonal relationships, or how these symptoms are manifested in particular contexts. She uses the DSM's vocabulary of the symptom-based descriptions, instead of more personal and detailed explanations of her emotions. For instance, she does not give us the contexts within which her "euphoria" or "manic state" arises, or the kinds of emotional states these terms refer to. She emphasizes the symptoms of her mood disorder over other components of her experience.

Consider the implications of this for Cheney's reasoning about her interpersonal relationships. She prefaces this part of her narrative by explaining it is not easy for her to establish long-lasting friendships with other women, because they do not accommodate her manic-depressive episodes. She says Linda, a friend in law school, was an exception, who according to Cheney, "weathered the bipolar storms with patience and understanding," and didn't get angry with her when she "was too depressed to call her back," or "cancelled long-standing plans over and over again" (Cheney 2009, 164). Note here that her perception of the success and failure of friendships is primarily attributed to her illness or people's responses to her illness, discounting other important factors that go into establishing relationships, such as character, compatibility, etc.

This hyponarrative framework also limited her responses to relationship problems. Despite her friendship with Linda, after she returned from ECT for her bipolar disorder, Cheney says she did something that is not typically tolerated in friendship; she started a relationship with Linda's boyfriend Jeff, while still "under the influence of the treatment." The relationship was initiated by Jeff; Cheney reciprocated in a mixed state of curiosity and guilt. Although she realized it is not acceptable in friendships to develop a relationship with one's best friend's boyfriend, she asked God:

> ...to consider the pleading circumstances: that between the mania-induced lust and the ECT-induced amnesia, I honestly forgot that there was anything more essential at stake, i.e., the unwritten rules of friendship. In particular, *Rule No. One: stay away from your best friend's boyfriend.*
>
> (Cheney 2009, 170; italics in original)

Importantly, in this passage, she refers to her psychological state at the time as "manic," linking her action to her illness, thereby circumventing her feelings of guilt. Looking at herself in the mirror, she says:

> That's when I knew: I owed my dear friend Linda allegiance, but I owed the woman in the mirror something more. It was miracle that I was still alive, after a year of bone-crushing, soul-starving depression. It was a miracle my brain still functioned well enough to flirt. I thought back to the face I'd seen in my bathroom mirror before the ECT: sullen, sallow, the smile muscles slack from disuse. And I looked at me now: pink-cheeked and blooming, trembling with anticipation, every pore, every freckle alive and alert. Funny I thought, I never pictured myself as one of "those" women—one of those heartless harpies who could steal a man right from under her best friend's nose. But try as I might, I just couldn't feel guilty. Much as I loved Linda, I realized now that my loyalties lay elsewhere. I owed it to myself to snatch at happiness however I could. Who knew when or if it would come again?
>
> (Cheney 2009, 172)

On the one hand, she ties her flirtation with Jeff to her mania, admitting her neglect of the consequences of her actions and the unwritten rules of friendships. On the other hand, she professes to be in love. Justifying her desire to get into a relationship with her best friend's boyfriend by referring to her unstable moods and manic state after the ECT is conflated with her acceptance of how much she feels connected to Jeff. Cheney writes, "It had to be love, I told myself. I wasn't the kind of girl who would betray her best friend for anything less" (Cheney 2009, 174). Although she tried to make it more than a "mania-induced affair," Cheney admits that after they broke up, the reality proved it was "mania," not "love." In the meantime, Linda was confused and disappointed as Jeff drifted away; she opened up to her friend. Cheney writes:

> A week, two weeks, a month went by, and Jeff and I grew closer every day. In all this time, I never once mentioned his name to Linda. She, however, kept bringing him up. She couldn't understand why he had suddenly pulled away. ... I'd murmur sympathetically, then talk of other things. But every day the guilt grew worse. I began to dread the telephone knowing that more likely than not the caller would be Linda, asking her eternal why. So I started answering less and less until eventually our conversations dwindled down once a week, then once a fortnight, then once a month, then not at all. I pleaded every excuse I could possibly think of to justify my silence: out-of-town visitors, a heavy workload, a recurrence of depression, the flu. But never once did I mention the actual truth.
>
> (Cheney 2009, 174)

Eventually, Cheney's friendship with Linda, as well as her relationship with Jeff, fell apart. Both incidents were upsetting for Cheney. She reports having feelings of sadness, despair, shame, guilt, and frustration, ending this section of the book, with the comment: "It's not about love, it's about retribution. When God wants to punish us, he grants us our sins" (Cheney 2009, 175).

What does Cheney's narrative about Jeff and Linda tell us? Clearly, parts of her writing display hyponarrativity; she separates the full complexity of her self-experience from her symptoms and excludes them from her story. In places, she considers her decision to begin a relationship with Jeff as arising from her manic state, separating what she, as a person, wants (to be in a relationship with Jeff) from her symptoms. Elsewhere, she reflects on her genuine interest in Jeff, finding him attractive, and so on. She oscillates between considering herself a whole person falling in love, albeit inappropriately, and attributing her decision to her symptoms and mania. She is confused about how she should be thinking about this and is left feeling guilty with no resourceful solution in sight. She has two failed relationships and mixed feelings about how and why they failed; at the same time, she is dealing with a mood disorder. Despite this complexity, the parts of her reasoning that deal with the challenges in her interpersonal problems pay more attention to the symptoms as explanations for the failed relationships.

Consider a couple of points here. First, although the starting point of her relationship with Jeff might be ECT-induced mania, Jeff's role in the relationship was important. Simply stated, discounting the latter and highlighting the former is not resourceful. Second, Cheney is not contemplating what the series of events leading to these failed relationships say about her mental health. Analyzing what happened, determining the roles of the various factors—especially the roles of Linda and Jeff—and seeing how her symptoms manifested themselves in the relationships might have resulted in understanding and self-insight. With an enriched degree of self-insight, for example, she might have talked to Linda. As someone who cared about Cheney and was familiar with her mood swings, Linda's feedback might have been helpful. Instead, Cheney avoided her.[2] This example illustrates the epistemic and ethical costs of twin failures.

3.5 Conclusion

This chapter examined the epistemic and ethical costs of sidestepping the self in contemporary scientific frameworks in psychiatry, with a focus on the Diagnostic and Statistical Manual of Mental Disorders (DSM). I argued treatment plans guided by the DSM framework fall short of being resourceful in guiding the development of effective interventions for patients. Similarly, patients' self-narratives shaped by the DSM framework sometimes constrain their responses to their experiences. The first part of the chapter explored the mechanisms through which the scientific frameworks in psychiatry shape the treatments patients receive and the way they think about their mental disorder, looking specifically at the mechanisms of the DSM's institutional and cultural power in clinical and personal contexts. The second part outlined the epistemic and ethical costs of sidestepping the self for flourishing.

Notes

1 Dennett distinguishes three "stances," or intellectual strategies, to make predictions about phenomena: the physical stance, the design stance, and the intentional stance. By adopting the *physical stance*, we can make predictions from knowledge of the physical constitution of the system and the physical laws that govern its operation. When we predict where a ball is going to land based on its current trajectory, we are taking the physical stance. By adopting the *design stance*, which is the domain of biology and engineering, we can make predictions based on knowledge of the purpose of the system's design (this could also be called the *teleological stance*). When we predict a bird will fly when it flaps its wings on the basis that wings are made for flying, we are taking the design stance.

2 My interpretation is not a personal criticism of Cheney, nor do I wish to undermine her account. Rather, I seek to show how a focus on symptoms might prevent a patient from responding resourcefully to interpersonal problems. In addition, this memoir reflects how the three factors might combine to influence a patient's response to interpersonal problems; it brings together the DSM hyponarrativity (focus on symptoms), DSM culture (self-diagnosis through self-help), and the individual's biased thinking (justifications to make sense of relationships).

References

American Psychiatric Association. 1994. *Diagnostic and Statistical Manual of Mental Disorders*. 4th ed. Washington, DC: American Psychiatric Association.

American Psychiatric Association. 2013. *Diagnostic and Statistical Manual of Mental Disorders*. 5th ed. Washington, DC: American Psychiatric Association.

Baylis, Françoise. 2011. 'I Am Who I Am': On the Perceived Threats to Personal Identity from Deep Brain Stimulation. *Neuroethics* 6, 513–526.

Cheney, Terri. 2009. *Manic: A Memoir*. New York: Harper Collins.

Dennett, Daniel C. 1971. *Intentional Systems*. *Journal of Philosophy* 68, 87–106. doi:10.2307/2025382.

Dickson, D.H. and J.W. Kelly. 1985. The 'Barnum Effect' in Personality Assessment: A Review of the Literature. *Psychological Reports* 57(1). doi:10.2466/pr0.1985.57.2.367.

Dmitruk, Victor M., Robert W. Collins, and Dennis L. Clinger. 1973. 'The 'Barnum Effect' and Acceptance of Negative Personal Evaluation. *Journal of Consulting and Clinical Psychology* 41(2), 192–194. doi:10.1037/h0035106.

Flanagan, Owen J. 1996. *Self Expressions: Mind, Morals, and the Meaning of Life*. Oxford: Oxford University Press.

Foo, Stephanie. 2022. *What My Bones Know: A Memoir of Healing from Complex Trauma*. New York: Random House Publishing Group.

Gigerenzer, Gerd. 2006. Bounded and Rational. In *Contemporary Debates in Cognitive Science*, edited by Robert J. Stainton, pp. 115–133. Oxford: Blackwell.

Gilbert, D. 2006. *Stumbling on Happiness*. New York: Vintage Books.

Gilovich, T. 1993. *How We Know What Isn't So: The Fallibility of Human Reason in Everyday Life*. New York: The Free Press.

Hacking, Ian. 1986. Making Up People. In *Reconstructing Individualism*, pp. 222–236. Stanford, CA: Stanford University Press.

Hacking, Ian. 1995a. The Looping Effects of Human Kinds. In *Causal Cognition: A Multidisciplinary Debate*, edited by Dan Sperber, David Premack, and Ann James Premack, pp. 351–394. Oxford: Clarendon Press.

Hacking, Ian. 1995b. *Rewriting the Soul: Multiple Personality and the Science of Memory*. Princeton, NJ: Princeton University Press.

Hacking, Ian. 1999. *The Social Construction of What?* Cambridge, MA: Harvard University Press.

Hacking, Ian. 2004. Between Michel Foucault and Erving Goffman: Between Discourse in the Abstract and Face-to-Face Interaction. *Economy and Society* 33(3), 277–302.

Hacking, Ian. 2007a. Natural Kinds: Rosy Dawn, Scholastic Twilight. *Royal Institute of Philosophy* 61(Supplement), 203–239.

Hacking, Ian. 2007b. Kinds of People: Moving Targets. *Proceedings of the British Academy* 151, 285–318.

Jopling, David A. 2000. *Self-Knowledge and the Self*. New York: Routledge.

Kahneman, D., P. Slovic, and A. Tversky. 1982. *Judgment Under Uncertainty: Heuristics and Biases*. New York: Cambridge University Press.

Lindemann Nelson, Hilde. 2001. *Damaged Identities, Narrative Repair*. Ithaca, NY: Cornell University Press.

Luhrmann, T.M. 2001. *Of Two Minds: An Anthropologist Looks at American Psychiatry*. New York: Vintage Books.

Lumsden, David. 2013. Whole Life Narratives and the Self. *Philosophy, Psychiatry, & Psychology* 20(1), 1–10.

Merkin, Daphne. 2009. A Journey through Darkness. *The New York Times Magazine*, May 6. www.nytimes.com/2009/05/10/magazine/10Depression-t.html.

Nguyen, Thi. 2024. Value Capture. *Journal of Ethics and Social Philosophy* 27(3), 469–504.

Poland, Jeffrey. 2001. Review of DSM-IV Sourcebook, Volume 1. *Metapsychology Online Reviews* 5(14).

Saks, Elyn R. 2007. *The Center Cannot Hold: My Journey Through Madness*. New York: Hachette Books.

Tekin, Şerife. 2010. Mad Narratives: Self-Constitutions Through the Diagnostic Looking Glass. PhD dissertation. York University.

Tekin, Şerife. 2011. Self-Concept through the Diagnostic Looking Glass: Narratives and Mental Disorder. *Philosophical Psychology* 24(3), 357–380. doi:10.1080/09515089.2011.559622.

Tekin, Şerife. 2013. How Does the Self Adjudicate Narratives?. *Philosophy, Psychiatry, and Psychology* 20(1), 25–28.

Tekin, Şerife. 2014a. The Missing Self in Hacking's Looping Effects. In *Classifying Psychopathology: Mental Kinds and Natural Kinds*, edited by H. Kincaid and J.A. Sullivan, pp. 227–256. Cambridge, MA: MIT Press.

Tekin, Şerife. 2014b. Self-Insight in the Time of Mood Disorders: After the Diagnosis, Beyond the Treatment. *Philosophy, Psychiatry, and Psychology* 21(2), 139–155.

Tekin, Şerife and Melissa Mosko. 2015. Hyponarrativity and Context-Specific Limitations of the DSM-5. *Public Affairs Quarterly* 29(1), 111–136.

White, Ruth. 2008. *Little Audrey*. New York: Farrar, Straus and Giroux.

Wilson, T.D. 2002. *Strangers to Ourselves*. Cambridge, MA: Harvard University Press.

Part II

Chapter 4

The Multitudinous Self

4.1 Introduction

This chapter develops a philosophically and empirically tractable model of the person—the Multitudinous Self Model (*MuSe*).[1] Grounded in research in naturalistic philosophy, cognitive sciences, and self-reports, the model is responsive to the experiences of "real people," as we encounter them in daily life, including those with or without psychopathology (Wilkes 1988). Remaining agnostic about the metaphysical nature of the self, *MuSe* provides a framework for systematizing the dynamic complexity of the self and its relationships with its physical, social, and cultural environments. Section 2 provides an overview of the philosophical and scientific approaches to the self that are reinvigorated through *MuSe*. Section 3 demonstrates how *MuSe* displays and organizes the complexity of the self by zooming into its physical, social, experiential, conceptual, and narrative facets. These have dynamic relationships with each other and with the physical, social, and cultural worlds. In addition, they allow the self to develop capacities for autonomy (the capacity and opportunity to make one's own decisions) and agency (the capacity to steer one's life in one direction or another). Through such processes, individuals construct their niche: they are not just shaped by their physical, social, and cultural environments—they also shape and transform them. It is important to highlight that these physical, social, experiential, conceptual, and narrative facets are not distinct parts of the self. Rather, they should be thought of lenses through which we can view the properties of the self. For example, we might think of the physical and conceptual facets of *MuSe* when we are trying to understand the athlete who lost a limb in an accident. We might say, "Losing their leg means that they can't play college basketball, and this has altered the way they conceptualize themselves as a competitive athlete." In other words, the facets of *MuSe* allow us to display and systematize the complexity of the self. Section 4 responds to skeptical worries about *MuSe* and highlights its pragmatic utility. This model, as will be developed in Chapters 5 and 6, can be a useful tool for psychiatry's fulfillment of its twin commitments: first, to arrive at

DOI: 10.4324/9781003055556-7

effective clinical interventions, and second, to enhance its scientific objectivity, while also offering resources for patients' own understanding of their mental disorders in a way that allows them to flourish. Thus, *MuSe* provides the conceptual and practical tools needed to link psychiatry's institutions with those touched by mental disorders.

4.2 Philosophy, cognitive science, and the self

The self is at once an exciting and controversial concept. Historically, philosophical approaches to the self have ranged from transcendental to deflationary views. On one end of the spectrum are transcendental approaches, developed by philosophers such as Plato, Aquinas and Descartes, who take the self to be a supernatural or metaphysical entity—the soul. Because the self is considered immaterial, it is not believed to be amenable to the mechanistic explanations found in the sciences. On the other end of the spectrum are deflationary views. Philosophers in this camp are skeptical about the self as a determinate thing, arguing it is nothing but a bundle of perceptions (Hume 1739), or a fiction, a center of "narrative gravity" (Dennett 1992), a myth (Metzinger 2009), or "mere social constructions" (Callero 2003). Yet the concept of the self plays a central role in sciences, including biology, immunology, sociology, and psychology, and care-oriented disciplines like social work. Given their pragmatic orientation, these disciplines make use of self-related concepts such as self-awareness and self-efficacy, especially in understanding how a human child develops, or in some cases, how psychopathologies emerge and can be treated. Unfortunately, this pragmatic literature does not precisely define what the self is, or what its mechanisms are. It is in this context of complexity and controversy that I develop *MuSe* in this chapter.

I am not a supernaturalist about the self; I don't think selves are souls or even that we *have* a "self." Nor am I setting out to convince the skeptic that the self exists. I am agnostic about the metaphysics of the self. Rather, my goals are pragmatic. I align myself closely with psychologists and empirically informed philosophers and make the case that it is conceptually and empirically plausible to talk or think about the selves we *are*. Selves have properties, including 1) physical properties, such as genotypes or appetite; 2) social properties, such as being a daughter; 3) experiential properties, for example, being disgusted by the smell of garbage; 4) conceptual properties, such as viewing oneself as honest; and 5) narrative properties, such as having a self-narrative about becoming a physician. These properties matter. They ground an individual's personal identity, in the sense of characterizing them as who they are, and they enable the individual to achieve their goals, connect to other people, develop agency and autonomy, and flourish.

Especially in the context of psychopathology, thinking about the self through its properties, as in *MuSe*, is resourceful. It allows us to make sense of the central properties of encounters with mental distresses or disorders, thus providing a target for scientific research, enhancing clinical interventions, and helping individuals to understand themselves and cultivate meaningful lives, notwithstanding mental disorder. *MuSe* displays the complexity of the self and systematizes it through its physical, social, experiential, cultural, and narrative facets, against the background of the physical, social, and cultural world. In developing the model, I follow in the tradition of psychologists, empirically informed philosophers, and feminist philosophers, such as William James, Ulric Neisser, Owen Flanagan, Bill Bechtel, Paul Thagard, Kathy Wilkes, Lorraine Code, Susan Brison, and Marya Schechtman.

Let me clarify what I mean by a model of the self. I use "model" in the sense of a "scientific model," which can be defined as a representation of an empirical phenomenon that facilitates access to that phenomenon for specific purposes. In science, models come in a variety of forms and employ different external representational tools, depending on the contexts in which they are used. Models can be objects, such as a toy airplane, or theoretical entities, such as Bohr's model of the atom (Bailer-Jones 1999). A model airplane might display the mechanisms responsible for an airplane's ability to stay in the air, and Bohr's model might illustrate the configurations of electrons and the nucleus in an atom, along with the forces acting among them. Model-building is a fundamental building block of scientific activity (Cartwright 1983; Hacking 1983). Models enable access to complex real-world phenomena by bringing forward certain aspects that make them amenable to manipulation and deliberately disregarding others in a process called "abstraction" and "idealization" (Godfrey-Smith 2006, 2009; Potochnik 2017). As a result, models tend to be partial descriptions or representations of a phenomenon. Model-builders select and identify relevant aspects of the target phenomena and use different types of models for different aims; for example, graphical models can visualize, and mathematical models can quantify the subject. In other words, models are developed with the goal of making them adequate for a specific purpose (Parker 2020). A model may sometimes have inadequate representational accuracy, but it may be just right when used for a particular purpose. Economists might use different models, for example, to represent the relationship between unemployment and gross domestic product, deciding whether to factor in or not factor in the inflation rate, depending on their purpose.

These commitments drove my development of *MuSe*. My goal was to represent at least some properties of the self in a way that is loyal to the selves or persons we encounter in our daily lives, with or without psychopathology. I aimed to represent the self in a way that displays its complexity while organizing and systematizing its properties so that the model can be used in contemplating and intervening in mental disorders. In other words, *MuSe* embodies my instrumentalism through and through, and it may or may not be useful in other contexts beyond mental disorders. However, I am not interested in exploring that possibility in this book.

A number of philosophical and scientific approaches to the self are implicated in *MuSe*. Their common denominators are their direct engagement with the relationship between the self and psychopathology, their embracing of patient experience in theorizing about mental disorders, and their attention to how cognitive sciences make sense of the self. My hope is that by rejuvenating these approaches, *MuSe* will help psychiatry redefine its relationship with science.

As discussed in Chapter 2, in the mid-twentieth century, the dominant framework for thinking about the mind or cognition was psychoanalysis, according to which mental lives are the products of the interactions between the conscious and unconscious of the mind. Freud's important contribution to the study of psychopathology was his case study methodology; he provided detailed accounts of his patients' mental distress, illustrating how the methods of psychoanalysis helped unpack their experiences and maybe treat them. Unfortunately, these case studies reflected more about the psychoanalytic assumptions about the mind than the real experiences of patients. Notably, Freud's patient Ida Bauer (named Dora by Freud) ended up stopping psychoanalysis as she felt Freud was imposing his own interpretations and theories about her past and psychological states on her, rather than giving uptake to her testimony (Moi 1981).

As Chapter 2 explained, psychoanalysis was subsequently challenged by behaviorism, according to which the best way to understand cognition is to study behavior. Behaviorism became the golden child of psychology and scientifically minded psychiatrists, as it helped develop empirical methods for investigating the mind by focusing on behavior. This led to a natural embrace of behaviorism and the medical model, in that leading biologically oriented psychiatrists took behavior to be an outward expression of underlying physiology, assuming biological interventions would help modify undesirable behavior by changing the physiology. This was also a ticket for psychiatry to establish itself as a properly scientific discipline, guided by Hempelian operationalism. Meanwhile, owing to the *Freud problem*, scientifically minded psychiatrists distanced themselves from any hint of psychoanalysis, falsely assuming any work on the human mind or the self would render psychiatry unscientific. Notably, the cognitive revolution in psychology, which developed methods for investigating the mind without subscribing to psychoanalytic notions like the unconscious or behaviorist notions like Pavlovian conditioning, was left out of debates on how to think of psychiatry as a form of science. I built on this thread of research in psychology and cognitive science of the self to develop *MuSe*, suggesting it will serve psychiatry's twin clinical and scientific goals.

One big influence on the development of *MuSe* in terms of both its content and method of development was William James. Beginning with psychology's recognition as a scientific discipline in the late nineteenth century, William James made major contributions to a picture of the self that he thought could plausibly be interrupted by the presence of a mental disorder. In his view, the self is constituted by four different but complementary selves: the material self, the social self, the spiritual self, and the pure ego. Psychopathology, he argued, such as multiple personality disorder, emerges when there are disruptions in these different selves (James 1890). James's approach was one of the first formulations of the naturalistic position in the philosophy of mind; he examined the nature of the mind in reference not only to metaphysics but also to the empirical sciences (Flanagan 1991a, 1991b), as well as the mental health- and distress-related experiences of well-known figures of his time (James 1902). For example, in *Varieties of Religious Experiences*, he takes Walt Whitman to be an example of "healthy mindedness," with a deep regard for "the goodness of life," (V 79) and a soul of "sky-blue tint" (V 80). He takes Leo Tolstoy to exemplify a "sick soul" by examining Tolstoy's "My Confession," taking what Tolstoy experienced as a kind of religious melancholy, as a state that could possibly lead to an experience of regeneration, being "twice-born." I will return to James's views as *MuSe* develops throughout the chapter.

Another formative figure in the development of *MuSe* was Ulric Neisser, the father of the cognitive revolution. Closely linked to the development of the computer, the emergence of the field of cognitive psychology in the 1950s and 1960s ushered in the cognitive revolution. With the cognitive revolution, psychology and cognate sciences of the mind distanced themselves from both psychoanalysis and behaviorism, arguing there *are* cognitive states *and* capacities of the mind, and they *are* prone to empirical investigation. So psychoanalysis was correct in supposing the mind had a structure, but misguided in assuming it was made of theoretical entities like the conscious and the unconscious, whereas behaviorists were wrong to argue that the mind did not matter, and only behavior could be studied scientifically. Cognitive scientists started studying cognitive processes scientifically, including perception, memory, attention, pattern recognition, problem-solving, language, and cognitive development, taking the computer as a model for the way human cognitive activity takes place and as a tool to specify the information-processing mechanisms that generate behavior.

Ulric Neisser was joined by Herbert Simon, Allen Newell, Noam Chomsky, and George Miller in spearheading the cognitive revolution. The publication of Neisser's *Cognitive Psychology* in 1967 ushered in this field of study. In this book, Neisser defines cognition as referring to "all the processes by which sensory input is transformed, reduced, elaborated, stored, recovered, and used" (Neisser 1967, 5). Going against behaviorism, he argues cognitive processes "exist, so it can hardly be unscientific to study them" (Neisser 1967, 5). Thus, cognitive psychology legitimized and connected a wide range of research paradigms in linguistics, anthropology, computer science, etc.

Neisser's later work guided both the content and the development of *MuSe*. In *Cognition and Reality*, Neisser advocates for cognitive psychology not to "confine itself to the laboratory and rely on computer modeling," but rather to "move to the real world and study how people act or interact in it" (Neisser 1976). By the same token, I believe theorizing about the selves and mental distresses or disorders should involve paying attention to the practice of psychiatry and mental healthcare and to the experiences and testimonies of people who are touched by mental distress and mental disorder.

Taken together, Neisser's four suggestions for cognitive psychologists serve as an ideal in my thinking about how *MuSe* must be regarded by those interested in studying mental disorders:

> First, cognitive psychologists must make a greater effort to understand cognition as it occurs in the ordinary environment and in the context of natural purposeful activity. This would not mean an end to laboratory experiments, but a commitment to the study of variables that are ecologically important rather than those that are easily manageable. Second, it will be necessary to pay more attention to the details of the real world in which perceivers and thinkers live, and the fine structure of information that world makes available to them. We may have been lavishing too much effort on hypothetical models of the mind and not enough on analyzing the environment that the mind has been shaped to meet. Third, psychology must somehow come to terms with the sophistication and complexity of the cognitive skills that people are really capable of acquiring, and with the fact that these skills undergo systematic development. A satisfactory theory of human cognition can hardly be established by experiments that provide inexperienced subjects with brief opportunities to perform novel and meaningless tasks. Finally, cognitive psychologists must examine the implications of their work for more fundamental questions: human nature is too important to be left to the behaviourists and psychoanalysts.
>
> (Neisser 1976, 7–8)

Note Neisser's emphasis on the methodology of studying cognition: paying attention to what people in the real world do, think, and perceive and developing theories and experiments that are ecologically valid, rather than running experiments that isolate individuals from their environment and giving them novel and meaningless tasks. Neisser invites psychology to turn its attention to the real world and real people. My goal is to resurrect these commitments of the cognitive revolution by putting the self at the center of inquiry in psychiatry.

In his later work, Neisser focused explicitly on the concepts of the self and self-knowledge, exploring the kinds of information that "specify" the self, i.e., the information we acquire that helps us develop knowledge about ourselves (Neisser 1988). He argued the forms of information that make us think we are a self are so different from each other that it is plausible to suggest each form of information establishes a different "self." Based on this argument, he proposed five selves: the ecological self, or the self that perceives and is situated in the physical world; the intersubjective self, or the self as a part of the social world who develops through interpersonal relationships; the temporal self, or the self in time who is grounded on memory and anticipation; the private self, or the self who is exposed to private experiences not available to others; and the conceptual self, or the self who represents the self to the self by drawing on the properties of the self and the social and cultural context to which it belongs. He investigated each of these selves by appealing to a wide range of work in cognitive science. He argued that even though the selves specified by five different kinds of information are not experienced as distinct, they differ in their developmental histories (e.g., the ecological and intersubjective selves start at birth, whereas the conceptual self develops parallel to the development of language) and in the psychopathologies to which they are subject. Thus, there is an explicit recognition that psychopathology is a property of the self. Alzheimer's disease, for instance, originates in the extended self but gradually influences the other selves.

Neisser's interest in the self led to the publication of various interdisciplinary collaborations with cognitive scientists and philosophers focusing on his different selves (e.g., Neisser 1993; Neisser and Fivush 1994; Neisser and Jopling 1997). This work exemplifies Neisser's own prescriptions for the field of cognitive psychology, in that it elaborates on the "selves" as we encounter them in the ordinary environment and in the context of their natural activities. It lays out the complexity of selfhood by considering its various aspects, for example, ecological, intersubjective, etc., as well as how the self systematically develops from infancy, how it perceives the environment and processes information available to it, how it interacts with others, how it remembers, and how it reconstructs experiences in remembering. This work is grounded in experiments in psychology and examines implications of the empirical research on the self to philosophical approaches to mind, self, and agency.[2] Near the end of his life, in his autobiography, Neisser says he "had high hopes that all this would have some impact on other people's theorizing about the self, but have seen little evidence of it" (Neisser 2007, 16). I hope this changes with the development of *MuSe*.

MuSe is also informed by philosophical work that takes seriously cognitive science and the experiences of individuals, including those affected by mental disorders. In an example of what I have previously called the "Real People Challenge" (Tekin 2020), Kathleen Wilkes argued philosophers of mind in the analytic tradition have much to gain from contemplating the experiences of "real people," including those experiencing what was then called multiple personality disorder (Wilkes 1988). As she was writing at a time when multiple personality disorder was popular among philosophers, Wilkes's approach was echoed by a range of philosophers (Dennett and Humphrey 1989; Flanagan 1991a, 1991b; Hacking 1996; Radden 1996; Tekin 2014a, 2014b). Similarly, important work has challenged the traditional accounts of agency by taking into account the experiences of "disorderly psychologies" and called for an empirically informed and pluralistic reflection on how persons develop agency and ethically order "the lives they live together" (Doris, 2015). For example, Jennifer Radden brought together the philosophical debates on personal identity over time and the research in cognitive and behavioral sciences to examine how people radically transform as a result of a mental disorder. For Radden, mental disturbances such as multiple personality disorder and delusions allow us to reconceptualize the traditional approaches to personal identity and abandon the notion of a bounded and unified self in favor of a view that posits a "succession of selves" (Radden 1996). This work aligns with feminist approaches to the self, according to which the self is not a disembodied, unified, bounded, and metaphysical substance, as the Cartesians claim it to be, but an embodied, dynamic, and relational entity responsive to the social and cultural layers of the community in which it is placed (Radden 2019; Willett, Anderson, and Meyers 2016). Radden suggested the normal or the typical self is heterogeneous and subject to variations and perturbations, and the psychopathological self must be understood in reference to it. Radden's work offers a rich framework to make sense of psychopathology in the context of typical human cognition, personal identity, and the self. It challenges the traditional conceptions of the self in philosophy and offers clinicians a framework for their treatment of individuals with mental disorders.

Another line of research influencing the development of *MuSe* involves the various kinds of scientific and philosophical work examining the connections between the self and the narratives about the self, that is, the stories individuals tell themselves about themselves (autobiographical narratives) and the stories others tell individuals about themselves (social narratives). Psychologists mostly use empirical studies of memory, joint reminiscence of the past, and parent-child narratives to examine how the self develops in response to autobiographical and social narratives (Fivush and Nelson 2006; Hoerl and McCormack 2005). Philosophers, however, often think of narrativity as having a temporal nature, whereby people remember the past and envision a future, or they situate themselves in a life-narrative. They use both thought experiments and real cases to cite experiences of mental disorders and connect them to the narrative nature of the self (Dennett 1992; Flanagan 1996). Some philosophers and psychologists take narratives or narrativity as merely *one* basis of personal identity and one cognitive tool used by the individual to construct self-concepts (Fivush 1994; Flanagan 1991a, 1991b; Tekin 2010, 2011, 2013). Robyn Fivush's work on parent-child narratives illustrates, for example, how social narratives shape children's perceptions and responses to reality, serving as a fundamental building block in their emotional development (Fivush 1998).

Others disagree, seeing narrative as *the* basis for self-constitution (Dennett 1991; MacIntyre 1981; Schechtman 1997).

4.3 The Multitudinous Self Model

As stated before, I am agnostic about the metaphysics of the self. *MuSe* takes the self to be a complex phenomenon in possession of various properties that connect it to the physical, social, and cultural environment in which the self is situated. *MuSe* integrates three bodies of information: philosophical work on the self, scientific work on the self and cognition, and first-person reports. By so doing, it aims to serve as a bridge between the sciences of the mind, individuals with experiences of mental disorders, and psychiatry, as will further be developed in Chapter 5. In this model, the self is world-directed and intentional (Dennett 1971), in possession of experiences (e.g., emotions such as disgust), mental states (e.g., beliefs, memories), and perceptions (e.g., smell). As a part of the physical world, the self has properties that enable it to maintain homeostasis and survive in the world. As a part of the social world, the self exists in relation to other social beings with varying degrees of regard. As a part of the cultural world, the self uses shared symbols, linguistic representations, and artifacts and hence shapes and is shaped by culture. Thus, the properties of the self allow for the evolutionary goals of survival and reproduction, such as developing and maintaining social relationships and learning, storing, and using information. All these enable the self to respond to—reflectively or unreflectively—its physical, social, and cultural environments.

Selves are complex and have many properties, but because of my present purposes, I take the self to possess the following properties: 1) physical properties, for example, genotypes, a cardiovascular system, blood type, etc.; 2) social properties, for example, being a daughter, a friend, etc.; 3) experiential properties, for example, feeling pain in a certain way, etc.; 4) conceptual properties, for example, being Canadian, honest, etc.; and 5) narrative properties, for example, having a self-narrative about becoming a doctor, etc. These properties are not independent; rather, they are in a dynamic relationship with each other and with the physical, social, and cultural environments. For example, properties of an individual's cardiovascular system shape and are simultaneously shaped by the individual's genotype, their parents' investment in their career as an athlete, their joy of playing basketball, their self-concept as a strong athlete, and their self-narrative as someone who wants to play like Kareem Abdul-Jabbar one day. Properties of the self and their interaction among themselves and with the physical, social, and cultural worlds allow the self to possess varying degrees of autonomy (the capacity to make its own decisions without interference) and agency (the capacity to act as a subject, making its own decisions, steering life in one direction or another).

To create pathways for the empirical investigation of the self, *MuSe* displays the properties of the self in a systematic way through five facets: physical, social, experiential, conceptual, and narrative. Facets of *MuSe* should not be thought of as "parts" of the self, as this is not an exercise in the metaphysical makeup of the self. Rather, facets of *MuSe* underline properties of the self that, once systematized, can allow the development of strategies that will help make sense of and intervene in mental disorders.

The *physical facet* includes the physical properties of the self, for example, genetic, hormonal, and neural properties that enable the self to perceive, respond to, and manipulate the physical environment. Thinking about the self through the physical facet of *MuSe* means learning about the physical properties of the individual whose self is in question.

The *social facet* includes the social properties of the self, for example, being relationally connected to parents, friends, or partners. Making sense of the self through the social facet of *MuSe* means learning about social properties of the individual whose self is in question.

The *experiential facet* includes the experiential characteristics of the self, for example, how the person experiences things from a first-person standpoint. This can be explained in reference to philosopher Thomas Nagel's argument addressing the limitations of reductionism in explaining consciousness. According to Nagel, each conscious organism has an experience of "what it is like" to be that organism (Nagel 1974). In a Nagelian spirit, the experiential facet provides information about "what it is like" to encounter the world. Making sense of the self through the experiential facet of *MuSe* means learning how the individual whose self is in question experiences themselves in the world.

The *conceptual facet* spotlights the properties of self-concepts, such as the ways the self views, thinks of, and represents itself. Self-concepts can be thought of as information-bearing units that underlie the beliefs individual hold about themselves. Examples of self-concepts are "being honest," or "being friendly." Making sense of the self through the conceptual facet of *MuSe* means learning what kinds of self-concepts the individual whose self is in question possesses.

Finally, the *narrative facet* underlines properties of the narratives the self creates about itself, in other words, the ways the self tells stories about its experiences in a selective and more or less sequential fashion. Making sense of the self through the narrative facet of *MuSe* means learning about the narratives the self creates and shares about itself, for example, wanting to be a physician since childhood, owing to many experiences at hospitals as a sick child.

4.3.1 Physical facet of MuSe

The physical facet of *MuSe* underlines physical properties of the self, which enable the survival, reproduction, and adaptation of the organism in a physical environment. Through various physical properties, the self perceives, responds to, and manipulates the physical environment.

Most processes underpinning the physical facet of *MuSe* emerge at birth and continue to develop and change in response to physical, social, and cultural environments. Some examples include the brain and nervous system, the endocrine system, the reproductive system, and metabolism and blood sugar. These systems are causally connected, and they make possible the interaction between the organism and the environment, enabling the individual to respond to, manipulate, and adapt to properties of the physical environment, such as climate, and to maintain homeostasis. Physical properties of the self that can be tracked through the physical facet of *MuSe* go beyond biological systems and include tools or artifacts that enable agency and coordinated movement (Neisser 1999). An artificial limb, or even a bike or a car, when actively used by the individual, should be characterized as a part of the self (Gibson 1979). Other features that can be examined through the physical facet include observable characteristics such as height or weight, skin color and complexion (e.g., white skin), sex assigned at birth, pregnancy, etc.

Note that the mechanisms underlying brain function or genotypes are among the properties of the self that can be understood through the physical facet of *MuSe*, but it is wrong to equate the self with the brain, part of the brain, or genotypes. Some scientists have given up the idea that "there must be some crucial center tucked away in some part of the brain that really is yourself" (Baumeister 2023, 5). In fact, some neuroscientists "have been so dismayed by this that they have concluded the self is an illusion" (Baumeister 2023, 5). Even so, there is significant body of research on the brain's default network system and its relationship with self-related thoughts (Tekin 2017; Yeshurun, Nguyen, and Hasson 2021). *MuSe* accommodates these various research threads; brain mechanisms, just like hormonal mechanisms, can be understood and studied through the physical facet of *MuSe*.

Properties of the self that can be traced through the physical facet are in a dynamic relationship with the other properties of the self that are trackable through the other four facets, and also with the physical, social, and cultural environments. All these properties and dynamic relationships co-constitute an individual's personal identity in the characterization sense: these features make individuals who they are (Schechtman 1997). As feminist philosophers have long argued, any reflection on selfhood must recognize that:

> "selves/subjects are always embodied and situated—which means always gendered, raced, and identified in various ways. To understand real selves, one needs to understand their particular positions and how, as such, they are thrown together into a complex, rich, challenging world."
> (Code 2006)

Another way of thinking about the physical facet of *MuSe* is to examine what William James calls the "material self," one of the five complementary selves discussed earlier:

> The body is the innermost part of the material Self in each of us; and certain parts of the body seem more intimately ours than the rest. The clothes come next. The old saying that the human person is composed of three parts—soul, body and clothes—is more than a joke. We so appropriate our clothes and identify ourselves with them that there are few of us who, if asked to choose between having a beautiful body clad in raiment perpetually shabby and unclean, and having an ugly and blemished form always spotlessly attired, would not hesitate a moment before making a decisive reply.
>
> (James 1890)

Here James is simultaneously addressing the physical features of the self and the way the person relates to those features. This is an important point in thinking about the physical facet of *MuSe*. The properties underlined by the physical facet can be accessed from both first-person and third-person perspectives. From the first-person standpoint, an individual directly perceives a bounded and controllable body; they see how their legs move when they are cycling, or they feel an itch in their arm, etc. Here James talks about the intimacy one feels towards one's own body—or clothes—and the value of these material properties on one's sense of who one is. From a third-person standpoint, properties underlined by the physical facet can be measured and investigated by others through either direct observation or scientific tools, for example, when a friend reports there is leftover food on our face, or when a clinician takes an X-ray of our knee. Both the first-person and the third-person points of view access the physical facet of *MuSe* and thus are important in understanding the physical properties of the self. An individual can reveal that they have a pain in their knee, and a physician looks at the X-ray to understand what might be underlying the patient's pain. Both ways of tracking the physical properties are needed to help the patient.

4.3.2 Social facet of MuSe

The social facet of *MuSe* represents the social properties of the self, such as being relationally connected to parents, friends, or partners. Social properties enable "species-specific signals of emotional rapport and communication" between the self and other people (Neisser 1988, 387). Most social properties emerge at birth and develop and extend over the life course as the individual interacts with others. In infancy, for example, the infant relates to immediate caregivers through an affective attunement mechanism. With the help of these social properties, the self relates to the social world in multiple ways: through one-on-one relationships of care, concern, and regard, and also through conflicts and disagreements. Social relationships give rise to social emotions of empathy and compassion, and through these emotions, the self may identify with others and operate as a part of that group or diverge from it and seek other social groups. The self continually adjusts itself to social expectations, it responds to social pressures and demands, and it seeks love and validation from others. Having lost a parent in one's teens, for instance, can be formative in one's character or habits of social connections. As James puts it, "the recognition" an individual gets from interpersonal relationships is fundamental for the self; humans are "gregarious animals" who have an innate tendency to be noticed favorably and to seek the respect of others:

> We are not only gregarious animals, liking to be in sight of our fellows, but we have an innate propensity to get ourselves noticed, and noticed favorably, by our kind. No more fiendish punishment could be devised, were such a thing physically possible, than that one should be turned loose in society and remain absolutely unnoticed by all the members thereof. If no one turned round when we entered, answered when we spoke, or minded what we did, but if every person we met "cut us dead," and acted as if we were non-existing things, a kind of rage and impotent despair would ere long well up in us, from which the cruelest bodily tortures would be a relief; for these would make us feel that, however bad might be our plight, we had not sunk to such a depth as to be unworthy of attention at all.
>
> (James 1890)

James is highlighting the intimate connection between the self and others; the self directly influences and is influenced by others. This codependency exists at the perceptual level—it doesn't need inference. For example, children may immediately perceive their parents are angry with them without having to make an inference based on their parents' behavior. Through such intimate relationships with others, first with primary caregivers and then the larger community, the individual's personal identity is formed, and their life can be enriched or impoverished depending on the qualities of these relationships. People who have been formative in our development, like our parents and siblings or our romantic partners, have the most influence on the social dimension of our self. In James's words, "The most peculiar social self that one is apt to have is in the mind of the person one is in love with. The good or bad fortunes of this self cause the most intense elation and dejection" (James 1890).

An important feature of the social facet of *MuSe* is its flexibility and dynamicity in response to the social world in which the self is situated. Selves can easily perform different roles and express different personality traits depending on the social environment. How we behave around our family is likely very different from how we behave around our colleagues. That does not mean the self who is with family is a different self from the one who is with colleagues. We simply show a different side of ourselves to each of these groups, depending on our joint history, rapport, and intimacy. As James puts it, we do not:

> "show ourselves to our children as to our club-companions, to our customers as to the laborers we employ. Many a youth who is demure enough before his parents and teachers, swears and swaggers like a pirate among his 'tough' young friends."
>
> (James 1890)

These different roles and identities work harmoniously, but at times, conflicts might emerge between different social properties of the self: the individual might feel shame or discomfort if a colleague sees them as they are when they are with family, or these roles "may be a perfectly harmonious division of labor, as where one tender to his children is stern to the soldiers or prisoners under his command" (James 1890).

Sociologist Erving Goffman highlights these features of the social facet of *MuSe* when he compares social life to a theater performance (Goffman 1959). In his view individuals "perform" their social selves according to the "stage" they take place in, i.e., the specific physical and social environment they are situated. Goffman outlines three stages for such performance, i.e., the "front stage" which refers to social contexts with a large audience that includes strangers, the "back stage," which refers to private contexts with a smaller audience comprised of people the individual knows, and the "off stage" when the individual is alone without any audience. Audiences in the "front stage" and "back stage" periods deeply shape an individual's performance, making the "off stage" a space where the individual can fully decompress, recharge and be authentic, without being subject to social expectations.

The social facet of *MuSe* can be understood from both first- and third-person perspectives. An individual might track their own social properties by examining the nature of their relationships and how they are in those relationships. For example, an individual might assess themselves as quiet and not very social around family, but more gregarious and interactive around others. Scientists such as sociologists can study the social facet of *MuSe* by observing individuals' social lives or using other scientific tools.

4.3.3 Experiential facet of MuSe

The experiential facet of *MuSe* highlights how the person experiences things as a subject. The experiential facet provides information about "what it is like" to encounter the world (Nagel 1974). The experientiality of the self makes our experiences uniquely ours. Our conscious experiences, including dreams, feelings, emotions, and sensations (e.g., feelings of pain or disappointment), are not phenomenologically available to anyone else, but with the help of language or other symbols (e.g., drawings) and other forms of representations, they can be communicated or shared (Bechtel 2007, 260). Through such sharing, we might discover others have similar experiences, or we may realize some of our experiences are unique. Consider reports of the sensation of the smell of onion, where one person describes it as "pungent." Others may find such a description illustrative of their own experience.

The experiential facet of *MuSe* emerges when children first notice they have direct access to their own experiences, and these are not shared by other people unless they tell them about these experiences. A child may realize, for example, that they are the only person who has a particular pain when they fall. While it is not certain precisely when children develop a sense of the privacy of their experiences, many studies show children are aware of the privacy of mental life before the age of five. For example, three- to four-year-olds locate happiness and fear in the action or object component of an event; six-year-olds, in contrast, locate the same feelings in the self, which is clearly appreciated as distinct from both objects and actions (Griffith 1992).

The experiential facet of *MuSe* is primarily tractable from a first-person standpoint. Individuals might report their experiences to others using language, or they may communicate the "what it is like"-ness of their experiences through other media such as drawing. However, in so far as experientiality is a property of *MuSe* that accompanies other characteristics of the self, such as its sociality, it is plausible to track the experiential facet based on third-person descriptions of one's experiences. My mother may tell a story about the time I got lost in the yard when I was a toddler. I am the one who experienced being lost, yet because of the immaturity of my cognitive capacities, a third person can provide a more reliable description of my experientiality. Finally, the experiential features of *MuSe* do not always align with reality. A teenager with a typical sized nose might experience themselves as having a big nose.

4.3.4 Conceptual facet of MuSe

The conceptual facet of *MuSe* highlights the ways the self represents itself to itself in the context of the physical, social, and cultural world. Self-concepts bear information about the self, enabling the formation of self-representations. In Roy Baumeister's words, self-concept is the "individual's belief about" themselves (Baumeister 2023). Self-concepts are formed in the process of dynamic interaction between the self and the physical, social, and cultural environments. Self-concepts include ideas and beliefs about our physical bodies (physical facet), interpersonal experiences (social facet), and our experiences (experiential facet) (Bechtel 2008; Jopling 1997, 2000; Neisser 1988). Self-concepts are derived from both the features of the self and the features of the physical and social environments.

For instance, an individual's self-concept as a "reliable person" is the product of the social properties of their selfhood and the norms of reliability in the culture to which they belong. Similarly, an individual's self-concept as a "short person" is based on both the features of their physical dimensions and the average height of individuals in their community. In that sense, I might have a concept of myself as a "short" person when I am in the United States, but consider myself a person of "average height" when I am in Turkey.

Self-concepts are not only representational but also edifying and action-guiding, as we compare our actual selves and our ideal selves (Tekin 2011, 2014a). This means self-concepts inform and shape the other dimensions of the self and are causally influenced by the changes the self undergoes throughout life. In other words, our actions help us move closer to our ideal selves in a process of self-concept development and maintenance. For example, if a person has a concept of themselves as an "unapproachable person" and feels this does not align with the kind of person they aspire to be, they may take steps towards being more approachable. Such change will require the person to adjust their social dimension; maybe they will start talking to a stranger on the bus.

Self-concepts are dynamic and plastic; they develop through childhood and early adulthood, when they are more easily changed or updated. With age and maturity, however, they become more stable and harder to change or modify. Self-concepts do not always align with reality. When they do, they are "congruent"; when they do not, they are "incongruent." Self-concepts vary from positive to negative, they have multiple emotional and intellectual functions, and they change according to the physical and the social context and over time.

The conceptual facet of *MuSe* is tractable from first- and third-person standpoints. From a first-person standpoint, an individual's self-reports can help us gather information about how they think about themselves. Similarly, from a third-person perspective, individuals' answers to questions, for example, about their self-efficacy, i.e., their ability to meet their own needs and lead a sufficiently independent life, are good ways to understand how they think about themselves.

4.3.5 Narrative facet of MuSe

Finally, the narrative facet of *MuSe* underlines self-narratives, i.e., the ways the self tells stories about itself in a selective fashion. Self-narratives are representations of complex states of affairs in an individual's life that selectively describe them in a coherent manner. In other words, they are cognitive sense-making tools which *selectively* connect, relate, organize, describe, and explain the states of affairs in the subject's life (Hutto 2007; Tekin 2011). By saying "states of affairs," I have in mind experiences, events, and relationships that weave the rich fabric of the subject's world. To give a few examples, the states of affairs in the subject's life include their ethnic background, their parents' occupation, the college they attended, the relationships they formed, the choices they made, the illnesses they had, the hallucinations they experienced, the tastes and habits they acquired, and so on. The activity of telling a narrative involves selecting and presenting these states of affairs to account for a component of the subject's world.

Self-narratives are multiplex: we can have narratives about various properties of ourselves. For example, self-narratives can be created based on our memories of our past, or our social life, or our physical appearance, or the evolution of our self-concepts. We simultaneously hold and share various self-narratives about our childhood, years in graduate school, our athletic abilities, the ways we think of ourselves, etc. They all co-exist and are sometimes congruent with each other and sometimes not. It is not implausible to think that an individual can have conflicting self-narratives about their childhood as being enriching and fulfilling thanks to moving around a lot while also being impoverishing and unfulfilling, owing to moving around a lot. It is part of the process of the cultivation of the self to try to adjudicate various conflicting narratives into more stabilized and consistent self-narratives.

The narrative facet of *MuSe* emerges later in life, usually after the physical and social facets, as the child starts developing episodic recall mechanisms, as well as language. For example, children as young as three have episodic recall. A two-and-a-half-year-old may fail to remember the particular "target event" an interviewer asks about but will have a fairly accurate memory at the age of three (Todd and Perlmutter 1980). Narrative capacities mature with time and play an important role in integrating the various dimensions of the self. Over time, individuals can reflect on their past experiences and future projections. Parent-child interactions, in which references to the past and expectations and anticipations for the future are rehearsed and practiced, are key to the maturation of this dimension.

Most people develop life narratives defining themselves in terms of a particular set of remembered experiences. Just like formal autobiographies, these accounts are not always accurate or unchanging, yet they are central to the way people think about themselves and guide their actions. Self-narratives do not always track reality, as they depend not only on the information once stored, but also on the social environment. There are cultural variations in the ways the self is connected to the past. The narrator of Marcel Proust's novel *In Search of Lost Time* is very concerned with the past and cannot escape its grip. The book features his recollections and examinations of his childhood and adulthood as a member of a high society in France. In contrast, philosopher Galen Strawson does not regard the past or recollections of it as self-defining, considering himself to be more "episodic" than "diachronic" (Strawson 2002).

The narrative facet of *MuSe* is empirically tractable both from first- and third-person standpoints; an individual can track the stories they tell about themselves, and others can track these narratives. From a first-person standpoint, some of these self-narratives are based on the recall of a childhood scene intimately available to the individual when, say, they smell a certain perfume that reminds them of their mother. This provides an anchor to the self-narrative. Language mediates the communication of self-narratives to others, opening them up to possible confirmation or disconfirmation and connected frictions, based on feedback from others. From a third-person standpoint, self-narratives can be qualitatively or quantitively examined using scientific tools. Similarly, just as we see in developmental psychology, narrative interactions between individuals can be studied scientifically. Finally, scientific examination of phenomena related to memory such as the connection between memory and the other parts of the limbic system can be central to this work.

4.4 Skepticism about *MuSe*

Skeptics might argue that the folk concept of the self does not sit well with the kind of concepts studied by the sciences, such as genetics and neuroscience, that promise to unpack the etiology of mental disorders and their mechanisms. This is why, they might suggest, the concept of the self is fractured into its different components, for example, memory, sense of self, etc., by those who study it. They may be skeptical about the ability of a model as complex as *MuSe* in terms of both its facets and levels of inquiry to do any important scientific work on developing interventions into mental disorders.

In fact, it is precisely due to the inscrutability of the self by science that researchers study the mechanisms underlying certain parts of the self. Skeptics may therefore argue the self is intrinsically private, and it is not plausible to conceive of scientifically generalizable regularities about it. They might be concerned that the phenomenal experience of the self requires "privileged access," whereby only the individual is a witness to their own mental states, and these mental states are not intersubjectively validated. For instance, how a teenager conceives their body (say, as overweight) is only directly given to them, not to others. Perhaps they falsely represent themselves to themselves as overweight; such a phenomenal experience cannot be intersubjectively validated. Others may perceive the teenager as within the normal weight range. Lack of an intersubjective validation of self-experience makes the concept of the self an unstable moving target, critics might argue. Similarly, some individuals with schizophrenia may report a deep sense of disintegration between themselves and their actions. Their bodies feel like alien objects; they feel they are automatons or machines, not agents who see, feel, eat, and suffer. Meanwhile, phenomenologically typical individuals are immediately aware that they are the subject of their feelings or actions, as they are simultaneously aware of said feelings. As philosopher John Perry puts it, for them, the self is the "unarticulated constituent" of experience (Perry 1998). If science aims at coming up with generalizable explanations and predictions of human behavior, how can it empirically track a self that appears to be intrinsically flexible, private, subjective, and accessible only to the subject whose self is in question?

In response to this question, critics might say scientists have been working on the scientifically tractable bits of the self, for example, the mechanisms underlying memory to develop interventions for Alzheimer's disease, or on identifying the brain mechanisms involved in disruptions of self-awareness in schizophrenia (e.g., the brain's default network system), and the role of genetics in the development of bipolar disorder. They might be skeptical about whether a complex model such as *MuSe* will get us closer to developing effective interventions for mental disorders.

Let's start with the challenge that a lack of intersubjective validation about self-experience makes the concept of the self an unstable moving target. It is true that there is a sense in which our experiences are only directly available to us, but this does not render the self an unstable or moving target. Rather, the goal of approaching the self through *MuSe* is to better display the complexity of the self and organize it in a way that makes (at least certain aspects of) it tractable by science. For example, the experiential facet of *MuSe* focuses directly on how the self experiences itself. As discussed above, our experiences are only directly accessible by ourselves, but with the help of language and other forms of representations and artifacts (e.g., art installations), they can be communicated or shared (Bechtel 2008, 260). Through such communication, we might discover that certain experiences are a part of our shared humanity (e.g., grief), while others are unique to us (e.g., extreme fear while driving). Thus, possible challenges in our intersubjective validation of our experiences do not make the self scientifically intractable; rather, they represent an opportunity to understand the complexity of the self and display it in a way that will render some of its features investigable by science. In addition, because *MuSe* aims to display and systematize the complexity of the self, its focus is not just on the experiential features of the self (represented through the experiential facet), but also on the physical, social, conceptual, and narrative facets. This allows, for example, at least some self-experiences to be evaluated using the other facets of *MuSe*, and in fact, such cross-analysis might illuminate certain features of mental disorders—this is important if *MuSe* is to be useful for responding to mental disorders.

Consider the example of how a teenager experiences their body directly as given to them, not to others. The teenager might perhaps have a self-concept as overweight. The experiential component cannot be intersubjectively validated by others, but the teenager might communicate to others how they feel, for example, while they are walking. Similarly, the conceptual component might not be intersubjectively validated unless the teenager spells out that they have a self-concept as an overweight person. However, through the physical facet of *MuSe*, using certain standardized measures such as the body composition metrics or the BMI, others (e.g., their doctor or their parents) might evaluate the teenager's weight as falling within the normal range. Through the intersubjective facet, their friends might state that the teenager does not look overweight, though the teenager might themselves be ashamed of their putative weight and stop socializing with their friends. This illustrates a discrepancy between how the teenager conceptualizes their body and how their body is perceived by others. Thinking about the teenager's relationship with their body, or even a connected eating disorder, through the facets of *MuSe* is resourceful. There is a window into how the teenager actually is and how they experience themselves, and efforts might be directed at helping them arrive at self-narratives that can engage with different properties of the self (grounded on both first-person experience and third-person observation) in a way that generates more congruency between their experiences and concepts, or that at least will allow them to develop skills to embrace these incongruencies in a way that can allow them to flourish.

This example also serves as a response to the second part of the worry, i.e., that working on the scientifically tractable parts of the self, such as memory, or brain mechanisms involved in self-awareness or genetics, might be more resourceful than studying this complex model of the self. I counter this criticism by highlighting the complexity of mental disorders. Mental disorders do not exclusively influence or change one property of the self. For example, the teenager's self-concept influences how they experience their body and how they relate to others socially. Studying a single property of the self alone will not 1) be helpful in understanding the full complexity of the experience of mental disorders; or 2) yield the rich results that will be effective in the development of interventions, the kinds that come from engaging with the mechanism of the self in all its complexity.

We gain a lot from looking at the self through the facets of *MuSe*. Properties underlined by each facet are in a constant dynamic interaction with the properties underlined by the other facets and also with the surrounding physical, social, and cultural environments. Individuals are shaped by these environments, but at the same time, they shape and transform them in ways that may facilitate or impede their flourishing.

Support for this view comes from the cognitive niche construction theory in cognitive science. This theory recognizes the centrality of environmental resources to human intelligence and suggests many organisms intervene in their environment and shape it in ways that improve the adaptive fit between the agent and its world (Sterelny 2010). Cognitive niche construction theory has roots in ecological niche construction theory, which states that organisms not only adapt to their environments, but also shape their environments, producing further adaptations. Berlotti and Magnani explain cognitive niche construction in the following way:

> Cognitive niche construction is the process by which organisms modify their environment to affect their evolutionary fitness by transforming their environment in ways that facilitate (or sometimes impede) the persistent individuation, the modeling, and the creation of cause-effect relationships within some target domain or domains. These modifications may combine with appropriate culturally transmitted practices to enhance problem-solving, and (in the most dramatic cases) they allow new forms of thought and reason.
>
> (Berlotti and Magnani 2016)

Cognitive niche construction happens on both the individual and the species level. Individual-level niche construction is relevant for *MuSe*. Through the properties of the self, underlined by the five facets, the self builds relationships with its physical, social, and cultural environments. In these interactions, the self develops capacities and traits that enable it to respond and adapt to these environments, while simultaneously shaping them. These interactions allow the acquisition of cognitive power and day-to-day problem-solving resources (Stotz 2010). Laland et al. emphasize the role of cultural processes in facilitating niche construction, arguing culture optimizes methods of passing down knowledge through teaching (Laland et al. 2012).

One possibly relevant extension of cognitive niche construction theory is Werner's concept of cognitive confinement (Werner 2019). Cognitive confinement occurs when someone is structurally or systematically unable to gain information from an environment, owing to a problem in their bond with their surroundings. Werner's main example is "filter bubbles" on the Internet that decrease the likelihood of obtaining new or unexpected information. This analysis can be connected to the analysis in Chapter 3 on how individuals adopt a medical stance by using DSM culture-based information about mental disorders to think about themselves and how this sometimes constrains their flourishing. In some ways, the DSM culture cognitively confines them to interpret their experiences from the lens of disorder and illness. Similarly, individuals such as Frame and Saks (see Chapters 1 and 2) could be said to have successfully constructed a niche that enabled them to flourish by helping them access to psychological, social, and cultural resources they needed to enhance their autonomy and agency.

Broadly stated, this is how *MuSe* illuminates the workings of the self in relation to physical, social, and cultural worlds. When the infant or the young child does not have fully developed properties, their needs are met by caregivers, and it is under the caregivers' guidance that the infant or the young child interacts with their physical, cultural, and social environments. During this time, they have limited agency and autonomy. As their physical capacities mature, the net of their social life expands, and their linguistic capacities develop. They start creating a conceptual world in which they form representations of who they are. They begin to develop self-narratives about themselves in relation to their physical, social, experiential, and conceptual facets which guide their actions and decisions. They grow increasingly independent from their caregivers, establish their own agency, and steer their lives in a certain way. As their agency and autonomy strengthen, they make certain choices about their bodies and their social life, adjudicating their self-concepts and self-narratives in the face of the values promulgated in their culture. In philosophical terms, the properties of the self are what characterize the self, making the self who it is. In Marya Schechtman's terms, the facets of the self provide information about the qualitative aspects of our lives (Schechtman 1997).

Thus, the properties of the self that are tracked by *MuSe* allow individuals to connect to themselves, their bodies, and their physical, social, and cultural environments. In typical circumstances, the interactions between the different properties of the self, as well as the interactions of the self as a whole with its physical, social, and cultural environment, are mostly coherent and seamless. However, the properties are not always aligned or congruent with one another. They may sometimes conflict and contradict each other, and they may clash with the physical, social, and cultural environments. For instance, through the information gathered by the social facet, I might be considered gregarious and friendly. It might be possible to track the number of friends I talk to on the phone on a given day or to list my social engagements on the weekend. Yet through the experiential facet, I might be construed as shy and introverted, based on my self-reports about myself.

Such inconsistencies or contradictions are typical; they simply illustrate that the selves contain multitudes. *MuSe* reflects these conflicts, as it draws on the multitudinous nature of the self, in the spirit of Walt Whitman's "Song of Myself" (1892). "Do I contradict myself?" asks Whitman, "Very well then I contradict myself / (I am large, I contain multitudes)." *MuSe* embraces the contradictions and inconsistencies within the self.

Admittedly, there can be inconsistencies and incongruences among the properties of the self that diminish an individual's agency and autonomy and flourishing. For instance, wars disrupt a soldier's self, and this can be tracked through the five facets of *MuSe*. Physically speaking, living under the physical circumstances of a war zone radically alters the physicality: from nutrition, to sleep, to being exposed to danger of being killed. Socially, watching one's fellow soldiers get hurt or killed disrupts the self. Conceptually, a soldier, once a good father and caregiver, intersubjectively/ socially defined as a compassionate and caring individual, may experience a serious disruption is these self-concepts after killing soldiers in combat, leading to a gap between their former and present self-concepts and destabilizing the balance. Similarly, a combat veteran may perceive themselves (falsely) as a coward after saving four out of five fellow soldiers, even though society may see them as a hero. The clash between information tracked through the five facets of *MuSe* might highlight inconsistencies and incongruences in an individual and cause problems. Such inconsistencies and contradictions might compromise an individual's agency and autonomy, cause their relationships with the physical, social, and cultural environments to deteriorate, and reduce their resources for flourishing. When thinking about what might help this soldier, tracing the properties of their experience with the five facets of *MuSe* would be a good resource.

Thus, *MuSe* simplifies the dynamic and complex nature of persons by drawing the contours of the self in a way that may make sense of the individual's encounter with mental disorders, thereby offering a pathway for the development of clinical interventions and enhancing flourishing. In other words, the properties of the self highlighted in *MuSe* can provide resources for the development of clinical interventions into mental disorders that will enable flourishing while enhancing the scientific rigor of psychiatry. In the next chapter, I explain how *MuSe* serves psychiatry's twin commitments to clinical effectiveness and scientific rigor.

4.5 Conclusion

This chapter developed a philosophically and empirically tractable model of the person—the Multitudinous Self Model, or *MuSe*—by engaging with research in naturalistic philosophy, cognitive sciences, and self-reports. Remaining agnostic about the metaphysical nature of the self, *MuSe* provides a framework for systematizing the dynamic complexity of the self and its relationships with the physical, social and cultural environments. Section 2 gave an overview of the philosophical and scientific approaches to the self that are reinvigorated by *MuSe*. Section 3 demonstrated how *MuSe* displays and organizes the complexity of the self by zooming into its five facets: physical, social, experiential, conceptual, and narrative. The properties of the self underlined in these facets have dynamic causal relationships with each other and with the physical, social, and cultural worlds. In addition, they all work together to support autonomy and agency. Section 4 responded to skeptical worries about engaging with the self through the five facets and highlighted the pragmatic utility of the model. *MuSe*, as I explain in Chapters 5 and 6, can be a useful tool for psychiatry to meet its twin commitments: to derive effective clinical interventions and to enhance psychiatry's scientific integrity. At the same time, it can offer resources for individuals to understand their own mental disorders in a way that allows them to flourish. Otherwise stated, the model links psychiatry's institutions with the people who are touched by mental disorders.

Notes

1 The inspiration for the name of the Multitudinous Self Model came from Walt Whitman's "A Song of Myself," from the lines, "Do I contradict myself? Very well then I contradict myself, (I am large, I contain multitudes.)" I am grateful to Owen Flanagan for helping me coin "Multitudinous," as the name of the model of the self I develop here and to Corey Maley for coming up with the best acronym I could imagine for the model, *MuSe*.
2 In her chapter "The Self and Contemporary Theories of Ethics" in *The Conceptual Self in Context*, Sheila Mason discusses the implications of empirical studies on the self and moral agency by considering three dominant approaches to moral theory in Anglo-American philosophy: the Rawlsian "justice model," the "communitarian model," developed by Alasdair MacIntyre, and the "ethics of care" developed by feminist theorists, including Carol Gilligan, Annette Baier, and Seyla Benhabib (1997). Mason argues Neisser's psychological theory of the self could be used to support the communitarian approaches to moral theory, as well as the approaches developed by the proponents of the ethics of care who highlight the features of the intersubjective self.

References

Bailer-Jones, Daniela M. 1999. Tracing the Development of Models in Philosophy of Science. In *Model-Based Reasoning in Scientific Discovery*, edited by Lorenzo Magnani, Nancy J. Nersessian, and Paul Thagard, pp. 23–40. Boston, MA: Springer.

Baumeister, Roy F. 2023. *The Self Explained: Why and How We Become Who We Are*. New York: Guilford Publications.

Bechtel, William. 2007. *Mental Mechanisms: Philosophical Perspectives on Cognitive Neuroscience*. New York: Psychology Press. doi:10.4324/9780203810095.

Bechtel, William. 2008. Mechanisms in Cognitive Psychology: What Are the Operations?. *Philosophy of Science* 75(5), 983–994. doi:10.1086/594540.

Berlotti, Tommaso and Lorenzo Magnani. 2016. Theoretical Considerations on Cognitive Niche Construction. *Synthese* 194, 4757–4779.

Callero, Peter. 2003. The Sociology of the Self. *Annual Review of Sociology* 29, 115–153.

Cartwright, Nancy. 1983. *How the Laws of Physics Lie*. Oxford: Oxford University Press.

Code, Lorraine. 2006. *Ecological Thinking: The Politics of Epistemic Location*. Oxford: Oxford University Press.

Dennett, Daniel C. 1971. Intentional Systems. *The Journal of Philosophy* 68(4), 87–106.

Dennett, Daniel C. 1991. *Consciousness Explained*. Boston, MA: Little, Brown.

Dennett, Daniel C.1992. The Self as a Center of Narrative Gravity. In *Self and Consciousness: Multiple Perspectives*, edited by Frank S. Kessel, Pamela M. Cole, and Dale L. Johnson. London: Psychology Press.

Dennett, D.C. and N. Humphrey. 1989. Speaking for Ourselves: An Assessment of Multiple Personality Disorder. *Raritan* 9, 68–69.

Doris, J. 2015. *Talking to Ourselves: Reflection, Ignorance, and Agency*. Oxford: Oxford University Press.

Fivush, R. 1994. Constructing Narrative, Emotion, and Self in Parent-Child Conversations about the Past. In *The Remembering Self: Construction and Accuracy in Self-Narrative*, edited by U. Neisser and R. Fivush, pp. 136–158. Cambridge: Cambridge University Press.

Fivush, R. 1998. Children's Recollections of Traumatic and Nontraumatic Events. *Development and Psychopathology* 10(4), 699–716.

Fivush, R., and K. Nelson. 2006. Parent-Child Reminiscing Locates the Self in the Past. *British Journal of Developmental Psychology* 24, 235–251.

Flanagan, Owen. 1991a. *Varieties of Moral Personality*. Cambridge, MA: Harvard University Press.

Flanagan, Owen. 1991b. *The Science of the Mind*. Cambridge, MA: MIT Press.

Flanagan, Owen. 1996. *Self-Expressions: Mind, Morals, and the Meaning of Life*. New York: Oxford University Press.

Gibson, James J. 1979. The Theory of Affordances. In *The People, Place, and Space Reader*, edited by J.J. Gieseking, W. Mangold, C. Katz, S. Low, and S. Saegert. London: Routledge, 2014.

Godfrey-Smith, Peter. 2006. The Strategy of Model-Based Science. *Biology and Philosophy* 21(5), 725–740. doi:10.1007/s10539-006-9054-6.

Goffman, Erving. 1959. *The Presentation of Self in Everyday Life*. Garden City, NY: Doubleday.

Griffith, Sharon. 1992. Young Children's Awareness of their Inner World: A Neo-Structural Analysis of the Development of Intrapersonal Intelligence. In *The Mind's Staircase*, edited by Robbie Case. London: Psychology Press.

Hacking, Ian. 1983. *Representing and Intervening: Introductory Topics in the Philosophy of Natural Science*. Cambridge: Cambridge University Press.

Hacking, Ian. 1996. The Looping Effects of Human Kinds. In *Causal Cognition*, edited by D. Sperber and A.J. Premack, pp. 351–383. Oxford: Oxford University Press.

Hoerl, C. and T. Cormack. 2005. Joint Reminiscing as Joint Attention to the Past. In *Joint Attention: Communication and Other Minds*, edited by N. Eilan, C. Hoerl, T. McCormack, and J. Roessler, pp. 260–286. Oxford: Clarendon Press.

Hume, David. 1739. *A Treatise of Human Nature*. London: Penguin Publishing Group, 1984.

Hutto, Daniel D. 2007. Narrative and Understanding Persons. *Royal Institute of Philosophy Supplement* 60, 1–15. doi:10.1017/S1358246100009589.

James, William. 1890. *The Principles of Psychology*. New York: Henry Holt, 1983.

James, William. 1902. *The Varieties of Religious Experience: A Study in Human Nature*. New York: The Modern Library.

Jopling, David A. 1997. A 'Self of Selves'?. In *The Conceptual Self in Context: Culture, Experience, Self-Understanding*, edited by U. Neisser and A. Jopling, pp. 249–267. New York: Cambridge University Press.

Jopling, David A. 2000. *Self-Knowledge and the Self*. London: Routledge.

Laland, Kevin N. and Michael J. O'Brien. 2012. Cultural Niche Construction: An Introduction. *Biological Theory* 6, 191–202.

MacIntyre, Alasdair C. 1981. *After Virtue: A Study in Moral Theory*. Notre Dame, IN: University of Notre Dame Press.

Mason, Sheila. 1997. The Self and Contemporary Theories of Ethics. In *The Conceptual Self in Context: Culture, Experience, and Self-Understanding*, edited by Ulric Neisser and David A. Jopling, pp. 233–248. Cambridge: Cambridge University Press.

Metzinger, Thomas. 2009. *The Ego Tunnel: The Science of the Mind and the Myth of the Self*. New York: Basic Books.

Moi, Toril. 1981. Representation of Patriarchy: Sexuality and Epistemology in Freud's Dora. *Feminist Review* 9(1), 60–74.

Nagel, Thomas. 1974. What Is It Like to Be a Bat?. *Philosophical Review* 83, 435–450. doi:10.2307/2183914.

Neisser, Ulric. 1967. *Cognitive Psychology: Classic Edition*. New York: Appleton-Century-Crofts.

Neisser, Ulric. 1976. *Cognition and Reality: Principles and Implications of Cognitive Psychology*. New York: W.H. Freeman.

Neisser, Ulric. 1988. Five Kinds of Self-Knowledge. *Philosophical Psychology* 1(1), 35–59. doi:10.1080/09515088808572924.

Neisser, Ulric. 1993. *The Perceived Self: Ecological and Interpersonal Sources of Self-Knowledge*. Cambridge: Cambridge University Press.

Neisser, Ulric. 1999. The Ecological Self and Its Metaphors. *Philosophical Topics* 26 (1/2), 201–215.

Neisser, Ulric. 2007. Ulric Neisser. In *A History of Psychology in Autobiography, Vol.* IX, edited by G. Lindzey and W.M. Runyan, pp. 269–301. Washington, DC: American Psychological Association.

Neisser, Ulric and Robyn Fivush. 1994. *The Remembering Self: Construction and Accuracy in the Self-Narrative*. Cambridge: Cambridge University Press.

Neisser, Ulric and David A. Jopling (Eds). 1997. *The Conceptual Self in Context: Culture, Experience, Self-Understanding*. Cambridge: Cambridge University Press.

Pamuk, Orhan. 2005. *Istanbul: Memories and the City*. New York: Knopf.

Parker, W. 2020. Model Evaluation: An Adequacy-for-Purpose View. *Philosophy of Science*, 87(3), 457–477.

Perry, John. 1998. Indexicals, Contexts, and Unarticulated Constituents. In *Computing Natural Language*, edited by Atocha Aliseda-Llera, Rob Van Glabbeek, and Dag Westerståhl. Stanford, CA: CSLI Publications.

Potochnik, Angela. 2017. *Idealization and the Aims of Science*. Chicago, IL: University of Chicago Press.

Radden, J. 1996. *Divided Minds and Successive Selves*. Cambridge, MA: MIT Press.

Radden, J. 2019. Mental Disorder (Illness). In *The Stanford Encyclopedia of Philosophy*, edited by Edward N.Zalta. https://plato.stanford.edu/archives/win2019/entries/mental-disorder/.

Schechtman, Marya. 1997. *The Constitution of Selves*. Ithaca, NY: Cornell University Press.

Sterelny, Kim. 2010. Minds: Extended or Scaffolded?. *Phenomenology and the Cognitive Sciences* 9, 465–481.

Stotz, Karola. 2010. Human Nature and Cognitive–developmental Niche Construction. *Phenomenology and the Cognitive Sciences* 9, 483–501.

Strawson, Galen. 2002. The self and the SESMET. *Journal of Consciousness Studies* 6(4), 99–135.

Tekin, Şerife. 2010. Mad Narratives: Self-Constitutions Through the Diagnostic Looking Glass. PhD dissertation, York University.

Tekin, Şerife. 2011. Self-Concept through the Diagnostic Looking Glass: Narratives and Mental Disorder. *Philosophical Psychology* 24(3), 357–380. doi:10.1080/09515089.2011.559622.

Tekin, Şerife. 2013. How Does the Self Adjudicate Narratives?. *Philosophy, Psychiatry, & Psychology* 20(1), 25–28.

Tekin, Şerife. 2014a. The Missing Self in Hacking's Looping Effects. In *Classifying Psychopathology: Mental Kinds and Natural Kinds*, edited by H. Kincaid and J.A. Sullivan, pp. 227–256. Cambridge, MA: MIT Press.

Tekin, Şerife. 2014b. Self-Insight in the Time of Mood Disorders: After the Diagnosis, Beyond the Treatment. *Philosophy, Psychiatry, and Psychology* 21(2), 139–155.

Tekin, Şerife. 2017. Looking for the Self in Psychiatry: Perils and Promises of Phenomenology-Neuroscience Partnership in Schizophrenia Research. In *Extraordinary Science and Psychiatry: Responses to the Crisis in Mental Health Research*, edited by J. Poland and Ş. Tekin, pp. 249–266. Cambridge, MA: MIT University Press.

Tekin, Şerife. 2020. Self and Mental Disorder: Lessons for Psychiatry from Naturalistic Philosophy. *Philosophy Compass* 16(1), e12715.

Todd, Christine M. and Marion Perlmutter. 1980. Reality Recalled by Preschool Children. *New Directions for Child and Adolescent Development* 1980(10), 69–85. doi:10.1002/cd.23219801007.

Werner, Konrad. 2019. Cognitive Confinement: Theoretical Considerations on the Construction of a Cognitive Niche, and on How It Can Go Wrong. *Synthese* 198 (7). doi:10.1007/s11229-019-02464-7.

Wilkes, Kathleen V. 1988. *Real People: Personal Identity Without Thought Experiments*. Oxford: Clarendon Press.

Willet, C., E. Anderson, and D. Meyers. 2016. Feminist Perspectives on the Self. In *The Stanford Encyclopedia of Philosophy*, edited by Edward N. Zalta. https://plato.stanford.edu/archives/win2016/entries/feminism-self.

Yeshurun, Y., M. Nguyen, and U. Hasson. 2021. The Default Mode Network: Where the Idiosyncratic Self Meets the Shared Social World. *Nature Reviews Neuroscience* 22(3), 181–192.

Chapter 5

The Multitudinous Self Model, mental disorders, and patient testimonies

5.1 Introduction

So far, I have argued the self has not been a target of investigation in contemporary psychiatry because of the *Freud problem*, i.e., a reluctance to engage with the self, owing to the strong association of the concept with psychoanalysis and worries about it weakening psychiatry's attempts to establish itself as a properly objective scientific discipline. Along with various other factors, this failure to investigate the self-led to the development of a psychiatric framework individuating mental disorders through observable properties such as signs and symptoms with the hope that their underlying mechanisms would be understood and addressed using the resources provided by the medical model. However, albeit inadvertently, the commitment to scientific objectivity came at the cost of hyponarrative conceptions of mental disorders that fail to engage with the thick complexity of patients' encounters with them and disregard their knowledge of their mental disorders in systemic knowledge production. These problems, which I have called psychiatry's twin failures, have effects on the clinical treatments patients receive and on patients' own reflections about and responses to mental distress and disorders, as documented in their self-reports.[1]

This chapter argues the Multitudinous Self Model (*MuSe*) provides new empirical and conceptual resources that enhance contemporary psychiatric practices, i.e., how mental disorders are understood and treated, by bringing to the fore previously underutilized or ignored sources of information about mental disorders. It does so, first, by conceptualizing what it means to have a mental disorder through the framework of *MuSe*, and second, by showing the indispensability of self-reports of individuals diagnosed with mental disorders in enhancing knowledge about mental disorders while also designing tools to organize and integrate such knowledge. *MuSe* helps us understand mental disorders in a way that rectifies the problems generated by the hyponarrative mental disorder descriptions prevalent in contemporary scientific frameworks. It also provides conceptual and empirical tools for engaging with mental disorders that are responsive to patients'

DOI: 10.4324/9781003055556-8

first-person experiences. Section 2 conceptualizes mental disorder using *MuSe* and provides a pragmatic distinction between mental distress and mental disorder. Section 3 examines why *MuSe* takes at least some patients as experience-based experts based on their self-reports and explains how it organizes the information gathered from them. Section 4 responds to the challenges to using self-reports as a source of knowledge in psychiatry. Once I have established how *MuSe* frames and engages with mental disorders and testimonies of individuals, in the next chapter, I show how the model can serve as a conceptual and practical tool to serve psychiatry's twin commitments to patient flourishing and to scientific objectivity.

5.2 *MuSe* and mental disorder

One of my motivations for developing *MuSe* was to decenter the labels for mental disorders in thinking about mental distress, mental health, and mental well-being, and similarly, to decenter the DSM as the only way various aspects of mental distress and disorder experiences can be managed. Thinking about mental distresses or disorders through the *MuSe* paradigm offers more resources for individuals and clinicians in making sense of and responding to individuals' experiences, as the focus is on the person as a whole, not on how their experiences may or may not fit a standardized diagnostic framework. The biggest resources of *MuSe* are its distinction between mental distress and mental disorder and its agnosticism towards metaphysical conundrums about definitions of disorder or disease.

In the *MuSe* framework, the concepts of mental distress and disorder are used pragmatically. "Mental distress" refers to an individual's felt unease or difficulty or psychological challenges, which raises tensions in their relationships with themselves and their physical, social, and cultural environments. There are many ways to manage mental distress, for example, exercise, better sleep routines, new friendships, travel, financial relief, new jobs, or medical interventions. If mental distresses are managed in the medical system, I take them to be "mental disorders." However, I do not use the concept of mental disorder as a metaphysical description that provides necessary and sufficient conditions for being a "disorder" and can be applied in every context. Rather, I use the concept of mental disorder pragmatically and circumstantially, reserving its use to individuate instances of mental distress that are examined and treated in medical contexts in contemporary health and disorder management systems. This means that to be considered as having a mental disorder, an individual must receive a medical diagnosis or treatment or must identify themselves as having a mental disorder by way of adopting a medical stance to make sense of their experiences, i.e., interpreting their experiences through the language of medicine. In other words, an individual's mental distress must *not* be considered a mental disorder in every context. In some contexts, it can be characterized as mental disorder to benefit from resources of the medical system that alleviate the distress; in other contexts, it can be characterized as distress so that non-medical resources open up. Or these two terms can be applied flexibly, depending on the context.

In any event, I think the concept of mental disorder is instrumental, pragmatic, and plastic. My goals in this book are pragmatic, and I am interested in how individuals encounter mental distresses and disorders and what they need from institutional structures, such as biomedicine or healthcare systems, in order to receive the support they need to flourish. I stay away from a universally applicable metaphysical notion of mental disorder. Instead, in my view, mental disorder is characterized instrumentally and is constrained to contexts of medicine or cases when individuals adopt a medical stance to make sense of their experiences.

Thus, not all mental distresses are mental disorders, but all mental disorders are mental distresses. A third category, "mental difference," includes individuals who consider themselves mentally different, but not necessarily as having mental distresses or disorders. Communities of individuals with autism serve as good examples. Some individuals in these communities identify their experiences as a form of distress; others see them as a form of mental disorder or a form of mental difference, and still others identify them as a permutation of the three categories. My focus in this book is on mental distresses and disorders; my arguments might have implications for mental differences as well, but I do not explore these.

I distinguish between mental distress and disorder for two reasons. First, my goal is to engage with the experiences of "real people" (Wilkes 1988), and I take these three categories—mental distress, mental disorder, and mental difference—to be representative of the experiences of many people. Second, I am interested in framing the experiences of individuals with mental distress and mental disorder in relation to the self for pragmatic rather than metaphysical reasons: I believe judgements about whether the experiences of a self or person should be classified as mental distress or disorder should be made for pragmatic reasons, in collaboration with the individual—to the extent that it is possible. I take both mental distresses and mental disorders to be potential constraints to flourishing, but whether they actually impede flourishing is contingent upon how they are addressed (not just by medical strategies, but also by other individual, social, or cultural strategies). Thus, it is very important that the ways individuals' experiences are framed enable them to have access to conceptual and empirical resources that will enhance their flourishing. This might mean, for instance, that one individual is classified as having a mental disorder in certain contexts and as having mental distress in others. For example, a teenager's distress surrounding the ability to stay focused could be categorized as attention deficit hyperactivity disorder (ADHD) to gain access to treatments such as medications and psychotherapy, while it might be prudent to present the teenager as having mental distress at school, so they do not falsely infer they will never improve, or to prevent them from being subject to stigma. In short, decisions on how to categorize someone's mental distress should be flexible and plastic, responsive to the needs of the self who is subject to the categorization.

My approach takes cues from Quill Kukla's radically pluralist, pragmatist and instrumentalist conception of disease and I apply it to my views of mental disorder. Arguing against a unified conception of disease, Kukla proposes an open-ended, pragmatic, and pluralist use of the concept and language of disease. It is appropriate to classify a condition as a disease "if (1) it is strategically helpful, with respect to some legitimate goal, to at least partly medicalize that condition or cluster; and (2) if within the epistemology and metaphysics of medicine, the condition or cluster can qualify as pathological" (Kukla 2022, 137).

My characterization of mental disorder embodies the "medicalization" part of Kukla's conjunctive account of disease, and I am not concerned, in the context of this book, with sorting out whether mental disorders are diseases in Kukla's sense. Rather, I use the concept of mental disorder in a way that medicalizes mental distress because it brings it under the "surveillance, management, and control of medicine" (Kukla 2022, 139). Here, following Kukla, I understand medicalization as having 1) institutional; 2) epistemological; 3) metaphysical; and 4) ethical dimensions. Institutionally, medicalization brings the topic of mental distress under the authority of institutions of medicine. When mental distress is medicalized, medical professionals become socially recognized experts who establish the standards for diagnosing a mental distress, managing it, and if available, providing treatments. Institutionally, clinicians use a variety of medical tools to track mental disorders and apply their knowledge and expertise to treating patients. For example, they examine the individual's behavior against the DSM diagnostic criteria for mental disorders. Epistemologically, medicalizing mental distress involves using the "tools, methods, and epistemic styles of medicine to understand and track it" (Kukla 2022, 139). Metaphysically, medicalizing mental distress involves "taking it as made up of the right sort of entities and processes to be tracked and understood using epistemic tools" (Kukla 2022, 139). For instance, under the DSM-style medical model, mental disorders are understood as a feature of the individual, not something that emerges in relation to that individual's social world. Ethically, medicalization of mental distress as mental disorder involves considering symptoms and signs as morally neutral, not a manifestation of bad character.

Calling an individual's experience mental distress or disorder can be resourceful or constraining, and I argue we should be flexible in our terminology, depending on the context. As Kukla highlights, medicalization comes with a variety of risks and potential benefits, and deciding whether it is strategically helpful to medicalize is often complex. Post-traumatic stress disorder (PTSD) was not considered a mental disorder until the publication of the DSM-III, and this categorization was damaging, as it prevented some veterans from receiving care for their mental distress upon returning from military service. In contrast, homosexuality was (wrongly) medicalized, and its classification as a mental disorder was limiting and constraining for individuals and impeded their flourishing. There are also conditions whose medicalization can simultaneously be beneficial and harmful, and this justifies choosing to call phenomena mental distress or mental disorder flexibly depending on the context.

MuSe can help adjudicate under which contexts it might be beneficial to medicalize mental distress by identifying an individual's mental distress as a mental disorder. It thus provides a conceptual and practical tool for clinicians, the individuals themselves, and their loved ones. The process under which such adjudication could be made would take the following form: when an individual encounters mental distress, the experience is examined through the facets of *MuSe*, i.e., physical, social, experiential, conceptual, and narrative facets, depending on the context and the reason for examining the individual's distress. This requires engaging with the physical, social, experiential, and conceptual facets to grasp the complexity of the individual's inquiry into mental distress and determine the resources they may need to address it. Each facet by itself and in relation to other facets will create different resources for both the individual and the clinician (maybe even the individual's loved ones) to address the individual's distress. These might involve calling the individual's mental distress a mental disorder so that certain benefits can be received, while others might involve not medicalizing the mental distress, such as, say, by helping the individual look for a new job. At the same time, a multi-faceted examination of the individual's distress will help them understand how their distress is influencing their relationship with themselves and their physical, social, and cultural environments.

Consider the following example. A 14-year-old records a TikTok video in which they report they are unable to sit still in the classroom, unable to stop fidgeting, and move around a lot. They say their parents and friends are frustrated with them for constantly interrupting them without waiting their turn. The teenager then reports their self-diagnosis as having ADHD. Suppose further that their parents see this TikTok video and disagree on whether the teenager is saying all these things to get attention (from friends or parents) or genuinely has a mental disorder such as ADHD, or a combination of both. The father says the teenager is fine; they are just like how he himself was at that age, and yes, they are a little too fast and too disruptive, but as they are a teenager, all this is fine, expected, and typical. He does not like that his child is self-diagnosing. He is worried about how the teenager's friends will treat them after seeing the video. Given the stigma of mental disorder, this public information might hurt the teenager's college entrance process if the selection committee somehow sees these public posts. The teenager's mother is worried and thinks her child has ADHD. She reports that she talked to teachers at school, and one teacher expressed concern about the teenager's overactivity and restlessness in class. She also shares that she Googled ADHD and read its symptoms, and she thinks the teenager definitely has it. The father says the teacher is exaggerating and doesn't understand what teenagers are like, whereas the mother thinks the teenager should be put on medication. They decide to get an expert opinion on what to do and how to address the teenager's mental distress and its social repercussions.

Let's say the clinician who is consulted provides an analysis of the teenager's distress via the physical, social, experiential, conceptual, and narrative facets of *MuSe*. For the physical facet, they will ask the teenager questions about their physical features, ranging from eating, sleeping, and activity habits to what they do at school. For the social facet, the clinician will ask about the teenager's relationships with parents, siblings, and friends. The clinician might further ask how their mental distress is influencing their relationships, or whether there are social situations in which their mental distress is heightened. When examining the experiential facet, the clinician will find out what the teenager feels like in their life at school, at home, and with friends and family. What is it like, for example, to feel restless all the time? What propelled the teenager to record that TikTok video to share their experiences? To understand the conceptual facet, the clinician will ask questions more broadly about what concepts the teenager would use to describe themselves and how they perceive themselves. Do they have self-concepts as a confident person, or not? What would the teenager think of themselves if they received an ADHD diagnosis? Finally, for the narrative facet, the clinician will ask questions about the teenager's life narratives, for example, what kind of narratives they have about who they are, what makes them who they are, or what they imagine their future to be like.

Engaging with all these facets will give information to the clinician that they might have missed if they only looked at the diagnostic categories provided by the DSM—it is concerned with observable behavior, not psychological states or personal narratives. In addition, they may recommend interventions that engage not only with the physical facet of the patient's self (e.g., ADHD medications), but also with social relationships, self-concepts, and self-narratives. In light of all these considerations, the clinician might explain to the teenager and their family that there are many unknowns about conditions currently labelled ADHD, and research on the subject is ongoing. However, they might add, an ADHD diagnosis might help the teenager be eligible for certain interventions covered by insurance that have been useful for other teenagers with similar conditions. The clinician may thus see it as appropriate for the teenager's distress to be referred to as a mental disorder, highlighting the pragmatic nature of this decision and emphasizing this label does not encompass all that might be going on. Given the information collected about the patient through the physical, social, experiential, conceptual, and narrative facets of *MuSe*, the clinician may also have other kinds of recommendations that might improve the teenager's physical complaints, experiential unease, social relationships, self-concepts and self-narratives. Engaging these facets, the clinician might choose not to characterize the teenager's distress as mental disorder and might recommend other ways of engaging with it. They might, point out, for example, that the teenager feels isolated and alone, as their parents are going through a divorce, and their recording of this TikTok video might have been a way to get attention. They may recommend that the parents show the teenager they still care about them even though they no longer want to stay married. The clinician, the teenager, and the teenager's loved ones can collectively or individually adjudicate which ways of framing and making sense of mental distress will help the teenager respond to their distress in a way that will allow them to flourish.

5.3 Self-reports and patients as experience-based experts

As we have seen in previous chapters, psychiatric knowledge of mental disorders and their treatment has traditionally been grounded in the DSM's conceptualization of mental disorders, the connected knowledge and research generated under the medical model, and the body of knowledge generated by psychiatrists' experience and encounter with patients over time. Most of the medical school and psychiatric residency education focuses on teaching trainees the DSM and medical frameworks, providing opportunities for them to observe practicing clinicians and psychiatrists as they interact with patients, and allowing them to treat their own patients under the supervision of senior physicians. *MuSe* expands the resources for psychiatric knowledge by adding a special epistemic space for self-reports in psychiatry's knowledge-building practices.

In a *MuSe*-based psychiatric epistemology, patients' self-reports play two roles. The first, as discussed in Chapter 4, is that *MuSe* systematically integrates and organizes information that comes from 1) patients' self-reports; 2) cognitive science; and 3) philosophy, none of which has received adequate attention as a source of knowledge in traditional psychiatric knowledge-building practices. Each of the physical, social, experiential, conceptual, and narrative facets of *MuSe* provides a way to frame what might be happening with the person with mental distress by taking into account their self-reports, alongside cognitive science and philosophy, in order to build a model of that person. In other words, *MuSe* systematizes the complexity of the self and thereby reveals how psychiatry can benefit from the adjudication of self-reports, scientific findings, and philosophy. The second role of self-reports in a *MuSe*-based psychiatric framework is to expand the notion of expertise to consider at least some patients as experience-based experts. As I establish in the next chapter, by so doing, *MuSe* enhances psychiatry's two commitments, first, to patients' flourishing, and second, to scientific objectivity.

Now, I want to examine how patients' self-reports are instrumental in considering at least some individuals with mental disorders as experience-based experts. As discussed in Chapter 2, the creators of the DSM explicitly turned away from the inclusion of patients in psychiatric knowledge-generation practices, arguing their inclusion would spoil psychiatry's efforts to arrive at scientific objectivity. In contrast, *MuSe* takes patients' participation as indispensable to knowledge generation, especially to develop interventions that enable flourishing and to improve the discipline's relationship with science. My contention is that at least some individuals with mental disorders who can express their experiences through self-reports could also contribute to psychiatric epistemology as "experience-based experts" (Collins and Evans 2002; Dings and Tekin 2023; Tekin 2020, 2022). This contention is grounded in an expansion of the traditional conception of expertise in science and the consideration of a range of factors giving an individual with the experience of mental disorder the knowledge and skills needed to be considered an experience-based expert.

A core question in philosophy of science and in science studies more generally is whether the public, specifically those individuals who are directly influenced by scientific research, should be involved in making scientific decisions, or whether decisions should be left to the experts trained in the relevant sciences (Collins and Evans 2002; Plaisance 2020). The goal in these debates has been to arrive at an equilibrium between a "problem of legitimacy," under which only a small group of individuals are seen as experts, i.e., those with specific training evidenced in degrees and certificates, and a "problem of extension," under which democratic motivations to build knowledge erase the gulf between experts and non-experts (Collins and Evans 2002). A solution to this debate has been the introduction of different categories of expertise in science (Collins and Evans 2002). The value of scientists' and technologists' knowledge and experience has been compared to the value of the public's knowledge and experience. In this new understanding, members of the public who have special technical expertise by virtue of "experience" are considered "experience-based experts," and as such, their contribution to knowledge production process is indispensable. The term experience-based experts refers to those whose expertise has not been recognized in the granting of certificates or degrees and highlights the centrality of experience. Experience, however, is not sufficient for an individual or group to be considered an experience-based expert. To become an expert in some domain, in this view, an individual must have direct experience *and* be embedded in the social life of the domain; in this way, they acquire tacit knowledge of fundamental states of affairs that pertain to the experience in question, and internalize central concepts, problems, and skillful actions to the point of fluency (Collins and Evans 2002). Experience-based experts contrast with other technical experts who have expertise by virtue of scientific degrees, certifications, or other credentials. This newer category of expertise enables pockets of expertise to be assigned to the citizenry and enriches the texture of scientific knowledge. The goal is to develop a discourse that will place their expertise alongside the expertise of scientists.[2]

A good example of experience-based expertise comes from Steven Epstein's *Impure Science*, in which he examines how, in the early days of the HIV epidemic, activists in San Francisco's gay community made indispensable contributions to the development of medical interventions (Epstein 1996). While these activists were not certified experts because they had not received appropriate training, they were experts by virtue of their direct experience with HIV and their interactions with the scientific and political community who made pivotal decisions about treatment. Specifically, Epstein says these activists developed "credibility" tactics by 1) acquiring a basic familiarity with the language of biomedicine to engage with the researchers; 2) positioning themselves as a stakeholder group representing the voice of all people with AIDS or HIV infection; 3) enhancing their understanding of scientific knowledge-building practices and drawing attention to practices that are not conducive to knowledge building; and 4) taking sides in pre-existing debates on how clinical research should be performed. For example, these experience-based experts pointed out that clinical trial subject groups consisted primarily of middle-class white men and argued clinical trial subjects must be representative of the entire population of individuals affected by the condition. They promoted a practical approach to conducting clinical research, one rooted in the needs and experiences of actual patients as opposed to an approach overly focused on abstract statistical analyses, as this approach may discourage AIDS patients from accessing care in trials. They demanded hasty approval of experimental treatments and established an organization that imported and distributed unapproved treatments for AIDS. Briefly stated, as experience-based experts, they worked to enhance knowledge-building practices in the development of AIDS treatments.

The framework of experience-based expertise is useful in highlighting the expertise possessed by at least some individuals encountering mental disorders who can formulate and share these experiences through self-reports. I argue patients who 1) have the experience of mental disorders and can articulate this experience using self-reports; and 2) who have learned from the experience over time with skill and effort (by carefully observing their own experiences as well as those of others), can be considered to have experience-based expertise on mental disorders. In other words, it is possible that some psychiatric patients may be able to acquire expertise through their own experiences and various treatments over time and also by observing other patients. Thus, patients with experience-based expertise can make positive contributions to psychiatric epistemology in general and to psychiatric science in particular. Especially in the context of the current crisis and controversy in mental health research, experience-based experts can offer unmatched resources to develop interventions that enable patients to flourish.

5.3.1 Current approaches to recognizing patients as experience-based experts

There is broad support for the view that at least some patients are experts by experience among some individuals diagnosed with a mental disorder. They consider themselves experts on a variety of dimensions of their condition, yet they articulate, correctly, that their expertise is rarely recognized as such. As an example, I quote at length from a memoir, *Musings of a Mad Activist,* written under the pseudonym "Borderline Academic":

> Every so often, I am told that I am "harping on my trauma" or "wallowing in self-pity" for speaking at length about the times I've been victimized. Much more often, and more benevolently, I am told that I am so "brave," or "bold" or "strong" for my willingness to be vulnerable and share personal details about my life. But it is very rarely, if ever, that I am treated as an expert. If I am treated as an expert, it is not because of my victimhood. It is because I am a PhD student, or an editor at a critical psychiatry web magazine, or a founder of a grassroots group that raises awareness about human rights violations. It is because of some position or title I have that is equated with productivity or empirical knowledge, with serving a population or doing work within the capitalist framework that is viewed as respectable, valuable, or most commonly, monetizable. The reality is that while all of the above experiences have contributed to knowledge about mental health, human rights, and cognitive liberty, it is deeply personal experiences of human rights violations and victimizations that gave me the bulk of my expertise. It is not study, readership, or editing that enables me to viscerally feel the impact of psychiatric coercion and paternalism in every bone of my body; it is not intellectual or empirical knowledge that drives me to speak out. It is only my subjective experience of victimization—which I feel and relive over and over each day—that leaves me with no choice but take action.
>
> (Borderline Academic 2019, 36)

Let me highlight a few elements Borderline Academic emphasizes about her encounter with a mental disorder, its diagnosis, and the ensuing medical and social treatment she received that make her believe she is an expert. To start with, her memoir reveals she has direct knowledge of what it feels like to have psychic pain. She also evaluates how she responded to different treatments, for example, hospitalization, and what may or may not have worked. In addition, she has a grasp of how her experience with mental disorder affects other dimensions of her life, such as her work and relationships. Finally, she is able to situate her experiences with the psychiatric and medical system in the larger context of human rights violations. Yet as she points out, she is never considered an expert on these issues by virtue of her direct experience; rather, when she is considered an expert, it is often because of her professional training. Borderline Academic's argument fits within a more traditional view of expertise, where someone is considered an expert on the basis of training and education; i.e., expertise is equated with technical expertise by virtue of one's knowledge of the subject matter on the basis of one's training. As she highlights here, she is not considered an expert on the basis of her encounter with mental disorder; the traditional notion of expertise excludes technical expertise by virtue of direct experience. She is recognized as an individual who is an expert because she *knows about* mental disorder, not because she *experiences* the phenomenon and demonstrates an understanding of her condition, its influence on her life, and the impact of various treatments.

Borderline Academic is not alone in highlighting the legitimacy of claiming to be an expert on one's own condition on the basis of one's direct experience with mental disorder, nor is she alone in expressing disappointment that she, as the subject of the experience of mental disorder, is not considered an expert by mainstream science (for some examples, see Boevink 2015; Lehmann 2015; Saks 2007; Tekin 2014, 2020; Tekin and Outram 2018). The number and quality of first-person memoirs of mental disorders wherein individuals report on their experiences and the medical and social treatment they have received have increased. While some individuals who write about their encounter with mental disorder are activists—many have become activists following negative experiences in the medical system—not all of them are. Some have written about their experiences for the sake of writing about them; others have done so because they want to make sense of their experiences in a sequential order, and still others want to share their experiences to help others with similar experiences. For example, William Styron's account of depression seeks to make sense of the change he encountered in his evolution from a person without depression to a person with depression and to understand the quality of his depressive states of mind. Similarly, Elyn Saks' memoir details how her encounter with schizophrenia evolved over time and how she benefited from or was harmed by different forms of treatment, such as psychoanalysis or DSM-oriented treatments. Wilma Boevink writes to provide a person-centric account of psychiatric ethics.

There are also movements such as the Mad Studies Movement, a psychiatric survivors' movement that is sometimes called a consumer/survivor/ ex-patient/service user movement. Movement members provide self-reports of their experiences for the purposes of activism and to raise awareness of the shortcomings of the medical systems wherein their distress has been managed. Growing out of the civil rights movement of the 1960s and 1970s, the early intellectual development of the movement drew on Judi Chamberlin's influential 1979 book *On Our Own: Patient-Controlled Alternatives to the Mental Health System*. The consumer/survivor/ex-patient/service user movement is not a homogenous group with clearly defined and shared goals and orientations, yet it generally pushes for justice, equitable rights, fair treatment, and destigmatization. It challenges the psychiatric system to stop taking an authoritarian approach and to work with service users to end systemic abuse. Among other things, it seeks to influence policy and to change laws that subject people to involuntary treatment (Chamberlin 1990; Oaks 2006). The consumer/survivor/ex-patient/service user movement exists to advocate for and give a voice to those individuals who have been marginalized based on their mental health condition. It is quite unlike other organizations with this mission, such the National Alliance on Mental Illness. These others are primarily composed of non-psychiatric service users, that is, psychiatric professionals and relatives of service users who "enthusiastically embrace the medical model" (Chamberlin 1990).

In my view, all these activists and individuals must be considered experience-based experts on mental disorders on the basis of their direct experience and the demonstration of their knowledge about these conditions and how they intersect with other aspects of their lives, as well as the social and cultural infrastructure they are embedded. Some argue there is an important distinction between memoirs written by activists and those by non-activists and suggest activism sometimes comes into conflict with knowledge building (see van der Vossen 2015). This is an important point, but I will not focus on it here. Rather, I believe all kinds of self-reports of mental disorder and distress are valuable in grasping the uniqueness of an individual's experiences, as well as the strengths and weaknesses of the ways they have been studied and treated both epistemically and socially. Each of these accounts provides a window into a phenomenon that is intrinsically complex. Sometimes, the writers of these self-reports can be considered experience-based experts.

In addition to patients and some clinicians, such as those advocating for patient inclusion in the DSM-5 (e.g., Sadler and Fulford 2004; Stein et al. 2010), increasing numbers of philosophers and psychiatrists are taking self-reports seriously and at least partly support the claim that some patients could be considered experts. In other words, there has been a participatory turn in philosophy of psychiatry, where individuals who are categorized under a certain label of mental disorder or disability are considered central to conversations about them. This can be characterized as being receptive to claims such as "nothing about us without us" made by individuals belonging to these groups (Catala 2020). Similarly, some philosophers advocate for taking self-reports of those who experience or witness mental disorders seriously in philosophical contemplation, especially those accounts available in the form of memoirs (Flanagan 2013; Tekin 2011, 2014, 2020; Tekin, Flanagan, and Graham 2017). For example, George Graham (1990) refers to J. S. Mill's experience with depression as a young man, notably how by probing his depression, he reached a deeper understanding of himself. Mill recognized the importance of aesthetic enjoyment and renewed his hope in his ability to change his character. In his case, Graham suggests, depression worked as a "recognitional epiphany in which he discovered certain truths and used them to shape his life" (Graham 1990, 417).

There is also increasing support for the claim that at least some patients must be considered experience-based experts. Philosophers have recently written about such topics as the role of self-advocacy activism in psychiatry (Arnaud and Gagné-Julien 2023), the necessity of including patients as experts in maintaining objectivity (Knox 2022; Tekin 2020), and the methods for involving patients as experts in a scientific psychiatry (Dings and Tekin 2023; Tekin 2022). Similarly, some have argued for the importance of involving experts-by-experience in the process of revising psychiatric diagnostic criteria (Fellowes 2023). In this sense, some authors promote amateur/citizen/user-led research conducted outside traditional academic settings by the mental health users themselves (Cooper 2017; den Houting et al. 2022). Similarly, a growing literature takes as its starting point the philosophical phenomenology of philosophers like Edmund Husserl and Merleau-Ponty and uses their views on human experience or the nature of consciousness to understand and examine the nature of the encounter with mental disorders. (e.g., Gallagher 2004; Parnas and Bovet 2014; Parnas, Bovet and Zahavi 2002; Maiese 2015; Sass 2010). At times, this body of work has directly shaped clinical work on mental disorders by way of developing clinical diagnostic scales to track the nature of self-experience and agency loss in schizophrenia (Parnas 2012). Work in this vein is now making an effort to connect more explicitly with a qualitative analysis of patients' self-reports (Ritunnano et al. 2022).

The idea of viewing patients as contributors to knowledge-building practices has wider reception in philosophy of medicine. Some philosophers advocate for the inclusion of patients' perspectives in medical case studies, noting their important contribution to medical epistemology (Ankeny 2017). A clinical case study, as a research methodology, is an empirical inquiry that investigates a medical phenomenon within its real-life context. Clinical case studies are based on in-depth investigations of individuals' illnesses to describe the details of a case, explore its underlying causes, study its unique aspects, create effective interventions, and so on. Ankeny says most clinical case studies are only presented from the physician's point of view; accordingly, "the doctor's voice becomes authoritative, even though in a sense his or her version of the events could be seen as a mere interpretation of the 'real' case as narrated by the patient" (Ankeny 2017). She argues for the inclusion of patient perspectives in clinical studies not just as a source of added value but also as a source of evidence, because patients provide unique details about their illness that may otherwise be overlooked.

Similar arguments appear in the medical humanities literature, in relation to medicine at large. In the last few decades, an important topic for proponents of humanistic approaches to medicine has been the nature of the relationship between the healthcare professional and the patient. There is a push to strengthen humanism in medical practice by encouraging medical professionals to recognize, seek, and engage with patients' narratives. Rita Charon, the founder of narrative medicine, argues the clinician must acquire the skills to listen to, interpret, and reflect on the patient's stories with an "engaged concern" to achieve therapeutic outcomes, because this is the fundamental way in which the patient learns to trust the clinician (Charon 2006). Narrative medicine focuses on the experiences of patients rather than on the generalizable propositions about them produced by logico-scientific inquiry. Active research and clinical programs in various hospitals are currently testing the fundamental tenets of narrative medicine in medical practice. Taking up patients' narratives is considered necessary not only to build trust between clinicians and patients but also to give physicians the means to improve the effectiveness of their work with patients, their colleagues, and the public. The *MuSe* framework for psychiatric epistemology that makes self-reports central to understanding mental disorders and promotes the view that at least some patients must be considered experience-based experts in generating psychiatric knowledge has a similar intent of humanism. A good way of enhancing psychiatric epistemology and practice is to give a voice to those directly affected by mental disorders.

Finally, important work is being done from the perspective of feminist philosophy of science, with researchers calling for the inclusion of patients' perspectives in the development of objective accounts (e.g., Gagné-Julien 2021; Tekin 2021). Some philosophers have started connecting the above-mentioned work to debates on epistemic injustice (Catala 2020; Crichton et al. 2017). While many common threads link the work on the value of first-person perspectives in psychiatric epistemology with the literature on epistemic injustice, philosophers of psychiatry have only recently started examining the direct connections between these areas of inquiry. It is my hope that the emerging work on epistemic injustice in the context of psychiatry and the anticipated experimental work on philosophy of psychiatry will present opportunities for cross-fertilization.

What has not yet been created is a methodology to integrate first-person reports and experience-based expertise in scientific, clinical, and reflective practices in psychiatry. *MuSe* represents a platform where all these sources of information can be systematically ordered and adjudicated. *MuSe* is able to integrate both self-reports and patients' expertise in knowledge-building practices in psychiatry by systematizing the information from self-reports through the five facets of the model and by considering at least some patients as experience-based experts who can enhance psychiatric knowledge.

5.3.2 Areas of patient expertise

Some patients, especially those who have been dealing with a chronic mental disorder for a long time, have a robust understanding of the *orientational challenges* associated with mental illness, such as psychic pain or other symptoms and signs of the illness. By orientational challenges, I refer to the "what it is likeness" (Nagel 1974) of an experience, for example, precisely how it feels when an individual has trouble getting out of bed (owing to low mood during depression), what it is like to have heart palpitations (during anxiety), or what it feels like to always believe their hands are dirty regardless of how often they wash them (during obsessive-compulsive episodes). Because such disruptions affect the total orientation of the individual and their relationship with themselves and with their physical, social, and cultural environments, they can be thought of as orientational challenges, in that the self has difficulty orienting itself in the world. Self-reports provide information on how such disorientation affects the individual's relationship with themselves and others. *MuSe* systematizes these experiences by tracking them through the model's five facets. For example, an individual might be experiencing heart palpitations in high-anxiety states (physical and experiential), and these might be intersecting with how they socialize with others; perhaps they are more withdrawn than usual (social) or conceptualize themselves as always nervous (conceptual) in their narratives about themselves, for example, "always feeling nervous before exams" (narrative).

In Chapter 1, I cited Janet Frame, who shares how she always felt different from others around her (experiential, social facets of MuSe). She explains the incident that led to her hospitalization when she was in a teaching practicum, why she suddenly left the classroom to never return (experiential, physical, narrative facets of *MuSe*). I also discussed Danquah, who writes about the dread she felt every morning trying to get up, explaining that taking care of her daughter was often her only motivation (physical, social facets of *MuSe*). Meanwhile, Brison describes how her body, which used to be a site for pleasure and a place to grow her own baby, suddenly turned into something that scared her after the sexual violence she was subject to, how cutting her hair was an instinctive way of protecting her body, her self (physical, experiential facets of *MuSe*). Finally, Knapp's descriptions of her cravings for alcohol are powerful and give us a grasp on what it is like to navigate the world in anticipation of the next alcoholic drink (physical, experiential facets of *MuSe*).

Some patients are experts on the *hyper-narratives* involved in the experience of mental disorder. In contrast to the hyponarrativity of the medical framework, their self-reports offer a thick and complex story of their personal experience. For example, we learn how the encounter with mental distress or disorder unfolds, how it emerges in the context of social relationships, possible age-related factors in its course, and how it shapes self-concepts and narratives. For example, the individual might report feeling uneasy and unsettled whenever they are at a gas station, and they do everything they can to avoid being exposed to the smell of gas. We might glean information by engaging with this person's self-report and systematize it by tracking their experience through the five facets of *MuSe*. We might find out, for example, that this individual is a Cambodian refugee, and the smell of gasoline causes distress (physical and experiential facets of *MuSe*) because it triggers memories of genocide (experiential and narrative facets of *MuSe*) during which the individual lost all their close family (social facet of *MuSe*). We might learn they have low self-esteem when it comes to driving because they really do not feel well when they are in the car (conceptual facet of *MuSe*). Through self-reports, then, we situate an individual's experience in the larger context of their life.

We also saw examples of this in Chapter 1. Frame contextualizes why she was considered different from others in relation to her family (social and narrative facets of *MuSe*), the poverty she grew up in (physical, social, narrative facets of *MuSe*). She talks about her insatiable thirst for writing and the dream of being a writer (narrative facet of *MuSe*) as she found her niche (narrative facet of *MuSe*). Similarly, Danquah takes us to her experience with depression in the context of her experiences as the child of an immigrant (social facet of *MuSe*) and her difficulty finding a community that she feels she belongs to in the United States (social, experiential, narrative facets of *MuSe*). She recalls how other Black women in her community did not believe her when she shared her depression experience (social facet of *MuSe*). In addition, the clashes between different cultures and norms, i.e., the assumption that as a Black woman she should be tough and just ignore things like her depression, as well as having a medical condition requiring a medical intervention, destabilized her self-concepts. She is in search of a narrative that is representative of her experiences; she questions "what color her depression would be" as a Black woman, referring to the framing of depression as a "black dog" in William Styron's descriptions.

Some patients are experts on the *therapeutic impact* of a psychiatric diagnosis. Individuals, especially those who have been in the mental healthcare system for a long time, have direct experience of a variety of treatment methods, ranging from psychotropic medications to psychotherapy and support groups. They can testify to the effects and side effects of medications and which ones were more or less useful in addressing their distress. From their self-reports, we glean information about the effectiveness of different kinds of psychotherapy; some may say they liked a supportive therapy, while others might explain why they benefited from Cognitive Behavioral Therapy. In other words, their self-reports give us a contextualized inventory of what has or has not worked for them in different circumstances, and these experiences can be systematically tracked through the five facets of *MuSe*.

We also saw examples of this in the first chapter. Elyn Saks compares the early diagnoses and treatments for schizophrenia she received under the psychoanalytic framework to the diagnoses and treatments she now receives under the contemporary DSM framework (experiential and narrative facets of *MuSe*). She also explains how the language used in the DSM to describe schizophrenia influenced her self-concepts and her visions for what her life might be like (conceptual and narrative facets of *MuSe*). Knapp describes how she eventually got better with the help of psychotherapy and by joining Alcoholic Anonymous (AA). Psychotherapy allows her to regulate her understanding of her past and her relationships with her parents (narrative and social facets of *MuSe*), and AA gives her a community (social facet of *MuSe*), accountability (conceptual facet of *MuSe*), and a niche.

Some patients are experts on *coping and flourishing* notwithstanding their experience of mental disorder. For example, most individuals who write memoirs featuring their mental disorders say the support they received from family and friends was crucial in the development of coping skills. Some note how relieved they were once they were diagnosed with a mental illness, because they were able to give a name to otherwise puzzling psychic experiences and seek others with similar experiences. Others say it was stigmatizing and dehumanizing to be reduced to a diagnostic label, and it prevented them from being part of a community.

Through a brief survey of a select number of memoirs and sociological research on mental disorder recovery rates in developing countries, my colleague Simon Outram and I found three factors seem to be especially important for individuals with mental disorder diagnoses to have a fulfilling life: 1) meaningful involvement in society and work; 2) participation in healing rituals in a community; and 3) levels of negative (or positive) expression about the individual with mental illness among family and community (Tekin and Outram 2018; see also Rosen 2006).[3] Information on what helps patients cope with mental disorders and flourish can also be systematized by looking at the five facets of *MuSe* in first-person reports.

First, consider the value of greater inclusion in the community and a fulfilling work role. In her memoir, Elyn Saks writes extensively about how studying philosophy and having a job that she loves helps her function and cope with schizophrenia:

> Everyone has a niche. Of course, resources are heavily skewed against the mentally ill, and the majority never have a chance to realize anywhere near their potential. ...I am not saying that everyone with schizophrenia or psychotic illness can become a successful professional or academic; I am an exception to a lot of rules, and I know that.
>
> (Saks 2007, 334)

What is key here, as Saks suggests, is that the individual find a line of work that is fulfilling, either financially or socially or both. Work satisfaction is an important aspect of her self-conceptualization and self-narratives. As such, this information coming from Saks's self-report can be catalogued using the conceptual and narrative facets of the *MuSe*.

Another patient, Ruth White, an assistant professor in social work who struggles with ADHD and bipolar illness, makes a similar point when she recalls facing serious challenges related to her mental disorders. She adds that what helped her reduce the disruptions of these experiences was the routine she created around work. She "never missed a day of work," as it gave her "something to look forward to, some sense of normality" (White 2008, 51). Her explanation can be categorized under the experiential, conceptual, and narrative facets of *MuSe*.

Mark Atkins, a professor of psychology and psychiatry who was diagnosed with schizophrenia and had hallucinatory experiences, makes similar arguments when he describes how he fully recovered from his condition by becoming integrated with a community through work. After leaving the psychiatric hospital, he volunteered at a local daycare center run by a regional school district and then was hired as a classroom aide. He later got a job there as a lead teacher and took extension courses on early childhood education. He says, referring to this transition from hospital to work, "Most remarkably to me, there were no racing thoughts and no depressive episodes or anxiety-laden interactions" (Atkins 2008, 183). Atkins's experiences can be consolidated using the experiential, social, conceptual, and narrative facets of *MuSe*.

Second, consider the role of participation in a community's healing rituals in enabling individuals to flourish. In their first-person accounts of dealing with mental disorders, many individuals mention their involvement in healing environments in a community. These include talk therapy sessions and support group meetings, as forms of healing rituals. The healing environments represent a type of extended kinship or communal network. They enable the individual to reflect on their self-experiences and feelings through a dialogue with others with similar experiences or with professionals who are trained to notice and engage with individuals' thought and feeling patterns. Involvement in healing environments in a community underscores the relevance and centrality of the social, conceptual, and narrative facets of *MuSe* in making sense of the circumstances that aid flourishing. In one memoir, the writer talks about going to an ADHD support group:

> [It was] the most amazing feeling. First, I was very uncomfortable with being in a group full of "sick" people. Even though I don't consider ADHD a "sickness." But I felt strange being in a support group. But at 8:30 P.M. when the meeting was over it was fabulous. To meet all those people who were like me. It was very "normalizing."
>
> (Hornstein 2008, 46)

Note that this individual's self-report brings out the social and the conceptual facets of *MuSe*; i.e., they are relieved to see other individuals with similar struggles, and they are able to conceptualize their self-experiences as more typical. In a similar vein, Saks suggests:

Medication has no doubt played a central role in helping me manage my psychosis, but what has allowed me to see the meaning in my struggles, to make sense of everything that happened before and during the course of my illness and to mobilize what strengths I may possess into a rich and productive life—is talk therapy.

(Saks 2007, 331)

Pointing to the benefits of this form of healing ritual, she adds, "People like me with a thought disorder are not supposed to benefit much from this kind of treatment, a talk therapy oriented toward insight and based upon a relationship" (Saks 2007, 331). As the memoirs make clear, talk therapy and group support meetings can provide a form of structured healing and offer an extended community, at least to some. And *MuSe* can help catalogue this information.

Third, a significant number of memoirs acknowledge the importance of a supportive family, information that can be catalogued through the social and narrative facets of *MuSe*. For instance, Atkins says, "My parents' and siblings' support … during those dark ages of psychiatric impairment, provided me with a strong foundation and confidence. There was always a place to return" (2008, 184). Positive family support helps patients build fulfilling lives. Some memoirs record high levels of negativity from friends and psychiatric professionals. These create a situation in which the individual is forced to respond to expectations of negative outcomes. A patient states, "I realized that once people know you're bipolar, they think everything you do is because you're bipolar" (Londahl-Shaller 2008, 276). He also says being identified with an illness becomes an expectation that your actions are all in relation to that illness—a form of negative re-enforcement.

Diagnosis appears to suggest patients should expect their lives to become significantly worse. Moreover, they cannot solve the problem or take remedial action to reduce the likelihood of this negative scenario. Worse still, they may feel an implied pressure to act out negative stereotypes. Thus, patients' orientational challenges include stigma and discrimination, exacerbating the difficulties in their lives. Ruth White talks about the reactions of her friends when she was diagnosed:

It was too difficult, too, for many of those same friends … to accept this new diagnosis. They questioned whether I was not simply stressed out from the many changes that had been going on in my life: a new job, a new city, my partner's move, and my new single-motherhood status.

(White 2008, 46)

To this, she adds:

Ironically some of my friends thought that I was just being over-medicalized and overmedicated. That angered me. For my friends to think that I was basically being emotionally lazy hurt me deeply. I knew that if I had called to say that I had cancer, the response would have been significantly different. I would have received empathy instead of being challenged on the validity of my diagnosis. ... I also understood that the change in diagnosis from ADHD to manic depression made them question the accuracy of my diagnosis, causing them to wonder whether I was just a victim of big pharma.

(White 2008, 46)

Thus, White's diagnosis led to a negative reaction from friends who questioned her diagnosis, which, in turn, was seen by White as questioning her judgement and moral qualities. Her friends appear to have been caught between accepting the diagnosis and seeing their friend as a form of human alien, or not accepting this diagnosis and risking alienating their friend by being unsympathetic. Either way, the diagnosis attracted strongly negative sentiments.

The engagement with self-reports and patients' direct inclusion as subjects of research can help us map how mental distresses interact with each facet of *MuSe* and develop multiple resources—not just medical ones—to aid flourishing, with or without the label of mental disorder. Specifically, *MuSe* provides tools to organize, systematize, and consolidate the information available in self-reports, so that it can be used by clinicians, researchers, and even individuals themselves. As I discuss in the next chapter, *MuSe* can be used as a repository of information on individuals' encounter with mental disorders while meeting psychiatry's clinical and scientific commitments.

5.4 Self-reports: Challenges and promises

5.4.1 Self-reports are not reliable

First-person testimonies or self-reports more generally have certain epistemic constraints. First, as philosophers have long argued, introspective reports do not always track truth and are not always reliable (Carruthers 2011; Schwitzgebel 2008). Challenging the Cartesian assumption that knowledge of our current thoughts is *infallible*, Carruthers argues such assumptions and the philosophical theories underpinning them are challenged by empirical evidence from across cognitive science (Carruthers 2011). For example, numerous psychological studies demonstrate how people *confabulate* their own thoughts, attributing thoughts to themselves that we have every reason to believe they never entertained (Gilbert and Wilson 2007).

In a classic paper "Telling More than We Can Know: Verbal Reports on Mental Processes," Nisbett and Wilson (1977) point out that we do not always have access to the cognitive processes underlying our actions, and they address some problems associated with using self-reports to study the mental processes of subjects. They suggest people can usually produce an explanation for their behavior when asked; however, their explanations may not be accurate because they may not have direct introspective access to all of their mental processes. Nisbett and Wilson review a number of studies supporting this claim. In these studies, subjects are placed in a context where they behave in a certain way. Their behavior is manipulated by means of an external stimulus. Subjects are later asked to explain their behavior. The explanation frequently does not involve the experimental manipulation. Subjects may report they were unaware of the stimulus or unaware that the stimulus influenced their response. In other words, people have a variety of mental processes for their preferences, choices, and emotions, but these may be inaccessible to conscious awareness.

Nisbett and Wilson contend introspective reports provide only an account of "what people think about how they think," not "how they really think" (Nisbett and Wilson 1977). Similarly, in a first-person narrative of mental disorders, the subject might provide an explanation for their actions without realizing the explanation fails to explain the actual causes of or motivations for their actions. In his later work, Wilson (2002) expands on this phenomenon, suggesting adaptive unconscious processes are highly involved in our cognitive processes. His use of the word "unconscious" goes beyond the Freudian concept of a repository of primitive drives and conflict-ridden memories. Unconscious processes, in Wilson's view, are sets of mental processes that implicitly pervade our mental lives, set goals, and initiate action, while we are consciously thinking about something else. He notes the difficulty of achieving self-knowledge through introspection only, because unconscious processes are responsible for many of our judgments, feelings, decisions, behaviors, choices, etc. In this view, self-knowledge can be attained by attending to unconscious processes, as well as the conscious narrative constructions of the self.

The lack of reliability in self-reports may also reflect the cognitive biases people employ when recounting certain events of the past. Individuals are found to have egocentric bias when they recall states of affairs; i.e., they remember past events in a self-serving manner (Ross and Sicoly 1979). For instance, students remember their exam grades as better than they were. A similar cognitive bias might be present in self-reports; subjects might reassess their past by representing themselves as honest, virtuous, and good, even if others have failed to see them that way.

Another example comes from Edward Jones and Richard Nisbett when they argue the actor's (i.e., the subject) understanding of the causes of their behavior does not necessarily conform to the understanding of outside observers (Jones and Nisbett 1987, 80), because the actor tends to emphasize the role of situational factors or environmental conditions while explaining the reasons for their actions. In other words, they appeal to the external causes of their behavior. In contrast, the observer explains the same situation by appealing to the actor's stable personal dispositions. Jones and

Nisbett suggest that this tendency often stems from the actor's need to justify blameworthy action, but may reflect a variety of cognitive factors other than the maintenance of self-esteem.

A self-report that focuses on the circumstances under which certain events took place will necessarily miss some aspects of the narrated states of affairs that would provide a detailed account of the subject's disposition. Jones and Nisbett note that in their autobiographies, former politicians report a perspective on their past acts which differs from the commonly held public perspective:

> Acts perceived by the public to have been wise, planful, courageous, and imaginative on the one hand, or unwise, haphazard, cowardly, or pedestrian on the other, are often seen in quite different light by the autobiographer. He is likely to emphasize the situational constraints at the time of the action—the role limitations, the conflicting pressures brought to bear, the alternative paths of action that were never open, or that were momentarily closed—and to perceive his actions as having been inevitable.
>
> (Jones and Nisbett 1987, 79–80)

These observations might equally apply to the reliability of self-reports, as similar cognitive biases may be at work. The subject may recount events in a way that emphasizes the circumstances, but this may differ from how others recount the same states of affairs.

While such skepticism on self-reports is sound, I do not think it warrants dismissing the value of self-reports in psychiatry. Whether or not they are faithful to the actual states of affairs in an individual's life, self-reports demonstrate the individual's perception of those states of affairs. In fact, these observations and perceptions provide a window into how the individual perceives their experiences with mental distress and disorder and their treatment by others, including medical professionals. Systematizing this information, without worrying about an absolute truth, will highlight properties of an individual's experiences that can be used to help develop effective interventions for clinical and personal use. In addition, as I explain in the next chapter, applying *MuSe* in clinical and personal contexts does not simply mean engaging with patients' self-reports; rather, it means using them systematically as a source of information in addition to the already used scientific and clinical knowledge about mental disorders, as well as research on the self in cognitive science and philosophy. *MuSe* provides a platform where all these diverse sources of information can be utilized to meet the goal of helping patients flourish.

5.4.2 Self-reports are hyponarrative

There may be a hyponarrativity problem with self-reports. I raised this issue in Chapter 3 in my discussion of the costs of hyponarrativity on individuals' reflections on their mental disorders. Self-reports reveal the *reflective impact* of psychiatric diagnoses, namely, how a diagnostic label affects the way individuals think about and understand themselves and how they adjust their self-concepts and self-narratives in response to a psychiatric diagnosis. In Chapter 3's discussion of the impact of DSM hyponarrativity on the way individuals think of themselves, I argued medical diagnoses can lead patients to take a medical stance towards themselves; i.e., they might interpret their self-experiences through the lens and vocabulary of medicine. This means an individual's mental distress is interpreted within a medical framework with a certain set of assumptions. Under the medical stance, which views mental disorders in the framework of the medical model, a person might believe they are experiencing mental distress because their brain is broken, and it can only be fixed with medications. Similarly, the TikTok teenager I mentioned earlier who self-diagnoses as having ADHD is adopting a medical stance, making sense of their experiences through the lens of the DSM criteria for ADHD. In any event, adopting a medical stance to understand and explain one's self illustrates the reflective impact of a psychiatric diagnosis. It influences the management of mental distress, say, by receiving medical treatments for ADHD, and serves as a way to conceptualize one's experiences and create self-narratives.

Note that adopting a medical stance is not always an active and deliberate choice by the patient; the way an individual's mental distress is framed and explained to them might become the only way they are taught to make sense of their experience. Consider what Wilma Boevnik writes about her relationship with her diagnosis:

> Until I learned about the concept of recovery as a journey, I was my disorder. I was provided with only one truth about my psychotic vulnerability and this was presented as the only truth. I was this devastating brain disease that could not be cured, and I would be limited more and more in my functioning in daily life. Never—during the years of my life that I was this ignorant, obedient patient—was I given alternative options for what happened to me. Neither did professionals, psychiatrists, around me know about alternatives. For them, their (medical) truth was the only truth.
>
> (Boevink 2015, 1)

She adopts a medical stance because that was the only stance she is taught. Terri Cheney's memoir (see Chapter 3) is similar. She adopts a medical stance to many of her problems in her social relationships, at the expense of evaluating them as problems of her relationships, not necessarily phenomena arising, owing to her bipolar disorder. We notice it in Stephanie Foo's memoir as well (See Chapter 3). After receiving the complex PTSD diagnosis, she uniformly thinks of her life through a medical stance, assuming all her choices and decisions are due to her PTSD. First-person testimonies like these illustrate how the reflective impact of a diagnosis could enhance or hinder flourishing.

Based on this, some may quite reasonably voice concerns about the reliability and helpfulness of self-reports in psychiatry. When self-reports draw on the available medical and scientific framings of mental disorders, it is hard if not impossible to discern what these individuals are actually experiencing. Otherwise stated, self-narratives may suffer from hyponarrativity, whereby individuals develop a tendency to adopt a medical stance to make sense of their mental disorder, thinking about their problems through the lens of a diagnosis instead of relating the broader contexts of their lives to each of the physical, social, autobiographical, private, and conceptual facets of *MuSe*. This might make self-reports irrelevant, some could argue, because they are simply relaying the existing medical accounts of mental disorders, not saying anything about patient's direct experience.

I have three responses to this challenge. First, just because some self-reports do not provide specific self-related aspects of the encounter with mental distress or disorder, we should not abandon their use. Writers of these memoirs are not a homogenous group, and the degree of self-reflexivity as well as the quality of writing can vary. Second, and more importantly, tracking the individual's adoption of a medical stance towards their experiences may give us information about how they conceptualize themselves and how they create self-narratives. With this information, we may be able to track the reflective impact of psychiatric diagnoses, including self-reflections that overuse the medical stance. This information could be systematically tracked in self-reports through the five facets, especially the conceptual and narrative facets, of *MuSe*. Such tracking can help us guide these individuals in developing a more resourceful way of thinking of their experiences. We can gently direct them towards reducing their medical stance and embracing other ways of thinking that may be more resourceful. Third, as mentioned in response to the reliability challenge, applying *MuSe* goes beyond merely engaging with patients' self-reports to include using them systematically as a source of information, in addition to the readily available scientific and clinical knowledge, not to mention the research on the self coming from cognitive science and philosophy. When taken together, these various resources serve as checks and balances and direct individuals' and clinicians' attention to metrics that will make a difference in patient flourishing.

5.5 Conclusion

This chapter outlined how the new empirical and conceptual resources provided by *MuSe* can enhance contemporary psychiatric practices, i.e., how mental disorders are understood and treated, bringing to the fore previously underutilized or ignored sources of information about mental disorders. Section 2 explored how mental disorders are conceptualized under *MuSe*, making a pragmatic distinction between mental distress and mental disorder. Section 3 examined why *MuSe* takes at least some patients as experience-based experts whose contributions to psychiatric epistemology are indispensable. Section 4 examined the challenges to using first-person reports as a source of knowledge in psychiatry and responded to them.

Notes

1 Recall that I use "self-reports," "first-person accounts," and "first-person testimonies" interchangeably.
2 Another useful category, "interactional expertise," refers to the ability to speak the language of a discipline in the absence of an ability to practice (Collins and Evans 2002). I believe interactional expertise is also a useful concept in the context of enhancing psychiatric knowledge, and interactional experts could help by establishing communication between experience-based experts and experts by training and also by providing a critical context in which these experts recognize and interact with each other. Philosopher Katie Plaisance proposes, for example, that philosophers of science can play the role of interactional experts and enhance scientific epistemic practices (Plaisance 2020).
3 Based on his research in developing countries, Alan Rosen suggests recovery from mental disorders is aided by: 1) social integration in the community so the individual maintains a status in society; 2) involvement in traditional healing rituals; and 3) availability of a valued work role that can be adapted to a different levels of functioning; (4) availability of an extended kinship, so family tensions and burdens are diffused, and there is low negatively expressed emotion in the family (Rosen 2006). In earlier work, a colleague and I mapped Rosen's suggestions to patients' memoirs (Tekin and Outram 2018).

References

Ankeny, Rachel A. 2017. The Role of Patient Perspectives in Clinical Case Reporting. In *Knowing and Acting in Medicine*, edited by Robyn Bluhm. London: Rowman & Littlefield.

Arnaud, Sarah, and Anne-Marie Gagné-Julien. 2023. The New Self-Advocacy Activism in Psychiatry: Toward a Scientific Turn. *Philosophical Psychology*, 1–24. doi:10.1080/09515089.2023.2174425.

Atkins, Mark. 2008. The Meaning of Mental Health (and Other Lessons Learned). In *Breaking the Silence: Mental Health Professionals Disclose Their Personal and Family Experiences of Mental Illness*, edited by Steve Hinshaw, pp. 175–189. Oxford: Oxford University Press.

Boevink, Wilma. 2015. Risk and Recovery: First-Person Account of Ethics in Relation to Recovery from Mental Illness. In *The Oxford Handbook of Psychiatric Ethics*, Vol. 1, edited by John Z. Sadler, K.W.M. Fulford, and Werdie (C.W.) van Staden. Oxford: Oxford University Press.

Borderline Academic. 2019. *Musings of a Mad Activist*. Edited by Andrew Collings. Published independently.

Carruthers, Peter. 2011. *The Opacity of Mind: An Integrative Theory of Self-Knowledge*. Oxford: Oxford University Press.

Catala, Amandine. 2020. Metaepistemic Injustice and Intellectual Disability: A Pluralist Account of Epistemic Agency. *Ethical Theory and Moral Practice* 23(5), 755–776.

Chamberlin, Judi. 1990. The Ex-Patients' Movement: Where We've Been and Where We're Going. *Journal of Mind and Behaviour* 11(3–4), 232–236.

Charon, Rita. 2006. The Self-Telling Body. *Narrative Inquiry* 16, 191–200.

Collins, H.M., and Robert Evans. 2002. The Third Wave of Science Studies: Studies of Expertise and Experience. *Social Studies of Science* 32(2), 235–296.

Cooper, Rachel. 2017. Classification, Rating Scales, and Promoting User-Led Research. In *Extraordinary Science and Psychiatry: Responses to the Crisis in Mental Health Research*, edited by Jeffrey Poland and Şerife Tekin, 197–220. Cambridge, MA: MIT Press.

Crichton, P., H. Carel, and I.J. Kidd. 2017. Epistemic Injustice in Psychiatry. *Psychiatric Bulletin* 41(2), 65–70.

den Houting, Jacquiline, Julianne Higgins, Kathy Isaacs, Joanne Mahony, and Elizabeth Pellicano. 2022. From Ivory Tower to Inclusion: Stakeholders' Experiences of Community Engagement in Australian Autism Research. *Frontiers in Psychology* 13, 876990.

Dennett, Daniel C. 1987. *The Intentional Stance*. Cambridge, MA: MIT Press.

Dings, Roy, and Şerife Tekin. 2023. A Philosophical Exploration of Experience-Based Expertise in Mental Health Care. *Philosophical Psychology* 36(7), 1415–1434.

Epstein, Steven. 1996. *Impure Science: AIDS, Activism, and the Politics of Knowledge*. Berkeley, CA: University of California Press.

Fellowes, S. 2023. The Importance of Involving Experts-by-Experience with Different Psychiatric Diagnoses when Revising Diagnostic Criteria. *Synthese* 202, 178.

Flanagan, Owen. 2013. Identity and Addiction: What Alcoholic Memoirs Teach. In *The Oxford Handbook of Philosophy and Psychiatry*, edited by K.W.M. Fulford, M. Davies, R. Gipps, G. Graham, J.Z. Sadler, G. Stanghellini, and T. Thornton, pp. 865–888. Oxford: Oxford University Press.

Gagné-Julien, Anne-Marie. 2021. Towards a Socially Constructed and Objective Concept of Mental Disorder. *Synthese* 198(10), 9401–9426.

Gallagher, Shaun. 2004. Understanding Interpersonal Problems in Autism: Interaction Theory as An Alternative to Theory of Mind. *Philosophy, Psychiatry, & Psychology* 11, 199–217.

Gilbert, D. and T. Wilson. 2007. Prospection: Experiencing the Future. *Science* 317 (5843), 1351–1354.

Graham, George. 1990. Melancholic Epistemology. *Synthese* 82(3), 399–422.

Hornstein, Gail A. 2008. *Agnes's Jacket: A Psychologist's Search for the Meanings of Madness*. New York: Rodale Books.

Jones, Edward E. and Richard E.Nisbett. 1987. The Actor and the Observer: Divergent Perceptions of the Causes of Behavior. In *Attribution: Perceiving the Causes of Behavior*, edited by E. E. Jones, D. E. Kanouse, H. H. Kelley, R. E. Nisbett, S. Valins, and B. Weiner, 79–94. Mahwah, NJ: Lawrence Erlbaum Associates.

Knox, Bennett. 2022. Exclusion of the Psychopathologized and Hermeneutical Ignorance Threaten Objectivity. *Philosophy, Psychiatry, & Psychology* 29(4), 253–266.

Kukla, Quill R. 2022. What Counts as a Disease, and Why Does It Matter?. *Journal of Philosophy of Disability* 2, 130–156.

Lehmann, Peter. 2015. Are Users and Survivors of Psychiatry Only Allowed to Speak about Their Personal Narratives?. In *The Oxford Handbook of Psychiatric Ethics*, edited by John Z. Sadler, K.W.M. Fulford, and Werdie (C.W.) van Staden, pp. 98–104. Oxford: Oxford University Press.

Londahl-Shaller, Esme A. 2008. He Just Can't Help It: My Struggle With My Father's Struggle With Bipolar Disorder. In *Breaking the Silence: Mental Health Professionals Disclose Their Personal and Family Experiences of Mental Illness*, edited by Steve Hinshaw, pp. 268–293. Oxford: Oxford University Press.

Maiese, M. 2015. *Embodied Selves and Divided Minds*. Oxford: Oxford University Press.

Nagel, Thomas. 1974. What Is It Like to Be a Bat?. *Philosophical Review*83, 435–450. doi:10.2307/2183914.

Nisbett, R.E. and T.D. Wilson. 1977. Telling More Than We Can Know: Verbal Reports on Mental Processes. *Psychological Review* 84(3), 231–259.

Oaks, David. 2006. The Evolution of the Consumer Movement: Comment. *Psychiatric Services* 57(8), 1212.

Parnas, Josef. 2012. The Core Gestalt of Schizophrenia. *World Psychiatry* 11(2), 67–69.

Parnas, Josef. 2012. DSM-IV and the Founding Prototype of Schizophrenia: Are We Regressing to a Pre-Kraepelinian Nosology?. In *Philosophical Issues in Psychiatry II: Nosology*, edited by Kenneth S. Kendler and Josef Parnas. Oxford: Oxford University Press.

Parnas, Josef and Parnas Bovet. 2014. Psychiatry Made Easy: Operationalism and Some of Its Consequences. In *Philosophical Issues in Psychiatry III: The Nature and Sources of Historical Change*, edited by Kenneth S.Kendler and Josef Parnas, pp. 190–212. Oxford: Oxford University Press.

Parnas, Josef, P. Bovet, and D. Zahavi. 2002. Schizophrenic Autism: Clinical Phenomenology and Pathogenetic Implications. *World Psychiatry: Official Journal of the World Psychiatric Association* 1(3), 131–135.

Plaisance, Kathryn S. 2020. The Benefits of Acquiring Interactional Expertise: Why (Some) Philosophers of Science Should Engage Scientific Communities. *Studies in History and Philosophy of Science* 83, 53–62.

Ritunnano, R., J. Kleinman, D. Whyte-Oshodi, M. Michail, B. Nelson, C. Humpston, and M. Broome. 2022. Subjective Experience and Meaning of Delusions in Psychosis: Systematic Review and Qualitative Evidence Synthesis. *The Lancet Psychiatry* 9, 458–476.

Rosen A. 2006. Destigmatizing Day-to-Day Practices: What Developed Countries Can Learn from Developing Countries. *World Psychiatry* 5(1), 21–24.

Ross, M., and F. Sicoly. 1979. Egocentric Biases in Availability and Attribution. *Journal of Personality and Social Psychology* 37(3), 322–336.

Sadler, John Z., and Bill Fulford. 2004. Should Patients and Their Families Contribute to the DSM-V Process?. *Psychiatric Services* 55(2), 133–138.

Saks, Elyn R. 2007. *The Center Cannot Hold: My Journey Through Madness*. New York: Hachette Books.

Sass, L. 2010. Phenomenology as Description and as Explanation: The Case of Schizophrenia. In *Handbook of Phenomenology and the Cognitive Sciences*, edited by S. Gallagher and D. Schmicking, pp. 635–654. Berlin: Springer-Verlag.

Schwitzgebel, Eric. 2008. The Unreliability of Naïve Introspection. *The Philosophical Review* 117(2), 245–273.

Stein, D.J., K.A. Phillips, D. Bolton, K.W.M. Fulford, J.Z. Sadler, and K.S. Kendler. 2010. What Is a Mental/Psychiatric Disorder? From DSM-IV to DSM-V. *Psychological Medicine* 40(11), 1759–1765.

Tekin, Şerife. 2011. Self-Concept through the Diagnostic Looking Glass: Narratives and Mental Disorder. *Philosophical Psychology* 24(3), 357–380.

Tekin, Şerife. 2014. Self-Insight in the Time of Mood Disorders: After the Diagnosis, Beyond the Treatment. *Philosophy, Psychiatry, & Psychology* 21(2), 139–155.

Tekin, Şerife. 2020. Patients as Experience-Based Experts in Psychiatry: Insights from the Natural Method. In *The Natural Method: Essays on Mind, Ethics, and Self*, edited by Eddy Nahmias, Thomas W. Polger, and Wenqing Zhao. Cambridge, MA: MIT Press.

Tekin, Şerife. 2021. *Towards a Socially Constructed and Objective Concept of Mental Disorder*. Presentation, Philosophy of Science Association Meeting, Baltimore, MA, USA.

Tekin, Şerife. 2022. Participatory Interactive Objectivity in Psychiatry. *Philosophy of Science* 89, 1166–1175.

Tekin, Şerife, Owen Flanagan, and George Graham. 2017. Against the Drug Cure Model: Addiction, Identity, and Pharmaceuticals. In *Philosophical Issues in Pharmaceutics: Development, Dispensing, and Use*, edited by Dien Ho, pp. 221–236. Dordrecht: Springer Netherlands.

Tekin, Şerife, and Simon Michael Outram. 2018. Overcoming Mental Disorder Stigma: A Short Analysis of Patient Memoirs. *Journal of Evaluation in Clinical Practice* 24(5), 1114–1119.

van der Vossen, Bas. 2015. In Defense of the Ivory Tower: Why Philosophers Should Stay out of Politics. *Philosophical Psychology* 28(7), 1045–1063.

White, Ruth. 2008. Finding My Mind. In *Breaking the Silence: Mental Health Professionals Disclose Their Personal and Family Experiences of Mental Illness*, edited by Steve Hinshaw, pp. 44–69. Oxford: Oxford University Press.

Wilkes, Kathleen. 1988. *Real People*. Oxford: Oxford University Press.

Wilson, Timothy D. 2002. *Strangers to Ourselves: Discovering the Adaptive Unconscious*. Cambridge, MA: Harvard University Press.

Chapter 6

The Multitudinous Self Model, flourishing, and science

6.1 Introduction

This book sets out to show that sidestepping the self in contemporary scientific frameworks in psychiatry has been costly for those diagnosed with mental disorders. As I explained in Chapter 2, psychiatry's efforts to develop clinical interventions that aid patients' flourishing while maintaining and advancing its scientific commitments has resulted, albeit inadvertently, in a mental disorder treatment framework that suffers from twin failures. First, in contemporary psychiatry, approaches to mental disorders are hyponarrativity, and the thick, self-related details of mental distress and disorder encounters are overlooked. Second, frameworks that aim to advance psychiatry's scientific commitment do not take advantage of patient expertise in knowledge-building practices in psychiatry. As a result, psychiatric care is at a stand-still, and the needs of individuals who experience mental distress and disorder are not met because available treatments are increasingly unable to help individuals flourish.

This chapter shows how the Multitudinous Self Model (*MuSe*) can be a resource to remedy these problems. More specifically, I argue the model can enhance psychiatry's commitments to both patient flourishing and scientific objectivity. It provides conceptual and empirical tools not just for clinicians to better support their patients, but also for the patients themselves, helping them strengthen their agency and autonomy. In addition, *MuSe* can help psychiatry realize its scientific aspirations by embracing more sophisticated notions of expertise and objectivity. Section 2 explores how *MuSe* can fulfill psychiatry's clinical and scientific aspirations by mobilizing the trilateral strategy, an integrative framework that relies on patients' experience-based expertise, scientific expertise, and clinical expertise. Section 3 shows how clinicians and patients can use *MuSe* and the trilateral strategy to enhance clinical resources and sharpen patients' reflective capacities to respond to mental distresses and disorders in a way that enables flourishing. As Section 4 explains, *MuSe* can improve psychiatry's relationship with science by offering a more sophisticated and expansive conception of what counts as

DOI: 10.4324/9781003055556-9

"expertise" and as "objectivity" in knowledge generation in psychiatry. Section 5 compares *MuSe* to the biopsychosocial model developed as an alternative to the medical model.

6.2 *MuSe* and the trilateral strategy

MuSe can meet psychiatry's clinical and scientific aspirations when used in conjunction with what I have previously called the *trilateral strategy* (Tekin 2016). While *MuSe* helps zoom into the self, the trilateral strategy helps zoom into the mental distress experienced by the self. The trilateral strategy is a methodological approach to examining an individual's mental distress (prior to decisions about diagnosis) drawing on three epistemic resources: 1) scientific knowledge grounded on psychiatry, medicine, and human sciences, such as cognitive science, sociology, and anthropology; 2) clinical knowledge grounded on training and know-how in psychiatry and medicine, as well as other care disciplines, such as social work, nursing, etc.; and 3) testimonial knowledge grounded on patients' self-reports. When combined, these three epistemic resources enhance the understanding of the particular mental distress in question and enable the development of strategies to strengthen the patient's agency and autonomy. For example, recall the case I cited in Chapter 5: the attempts to make sense of the teenager's attention-related concerns. Using a trilateral strategy to examine attention-related problems in this context would mean putting together 1) scientific knowledge on attention as a cognitive function; 2) clinical knowledge on attention-related disorders and interventions that have or have not been helpful for teenagers; and 3) testimonial knowledge grounded on the self-reports of individuals who have encountered attention-related distresses and disorders, acquired by reading memoirs, blogs, interviews, etc.

Using *MuSe* in conjunction with the trilateral strategy looks like following. Suppose a person with mental distress becomes an object of investigation for an investigator—whether a clinician, the individual themselves, or a scientist. The first step for the investigator is to draw a picture of the individual through the five facets of *MuSe*, i.e., the physical, social, experiential, conceptual, and narrative facets of the individual. The second step is to mobilize the trilateral strategy to draw a picture of the mental distress the individual is experiencing, by referring to the relevant scientific, clinical, and testimonial knowledge. Juxtaposing the information about the individual gathered through *MuSe* to the information about the mental distress gathered through the trilateral strategy will provide a philosophically and empirically informed assessment of the individual's encounter with mental distress, leading, for example, the clinician to label it a mental disorder, if this is thought to benefit the individual. As discussed in the previous chapter, this assessment will be made based on the instrumental value of a mental disorder categorization and will be used flexibly, depending on the context.

Using *MuSe* in conjunction with the trilateral strategy will enable the clinician to customize interventional strategies to address this particular individual's mental distress/disorder. This means that in addition to resources provided by psychiatry and medicine, the clinician will be able to utilize the resources of cognitive science, psychology, and even philosophy, in, say, understanding the features of the individual's encounter with mental distress and its relationship to the individual's personal identity, social relationships, work status, self-concepts, etc. and helping the individual access practical and conceptual resources that will enable them to act in a way that strengthens their agency and autonomy.

The use of *MuSe* in conjunction with the trilateral strategy can provide resources for psychiatry that have previously been underutilized, including: testimonial knowledge derived from patients' self-reports and experience-based expertise; scientific knowledge provided by human sciences, such as cognitive science, psychology, anthropology, and sociology; clinical knowledge derived from care disciplines such as social work or clinical psychology; and philosophical approaches to the self that provide conceptual tools for engaging with the different aspects of self-experience and flourishing. While relying on the scientific and clinical expertise of psychiatrists to examine and treat mental disorders is *modus operandi* in contemporary psychiatry, drawing on the above-mentioned resources is not, and this is costly, especially for developing interventions that enable flourishing.

Consider testimonial knowledge. As discussed in Chapter 5, we now have access to many self-reports of the experience of mental distress and disorder, and at least some patients who have written about their experiences can be considered to have experience-based expertise on mental disorders. Thus, these individuals can provide valuable insights into various aspects of living with a mental disorder, from orientational challenges to developing coping skills and creating a personal niche. They have much to offer in understanding and addressing psychopathology. Despite this, as I have established, experience-based experts are not made part of the knowledge-building practices in psychiatry, nor is engaging with testimonial knowledge encouraged in medical education or clinical training. The use of *MuSe* in conjunction with the trilateral strategy enables access to the underutilized testimonial knowledge.

Consider next the research in the human sciences. As highlighted in Chapter 2, since the 1980s, research and funding priorities in psychiatry have been skewed towards the biological sciences, with increased funding of projects in genetics and neuroscience. The scientific knowledge originating in the human sciences, such as psychology, cognitive science, sociology, and anthropology, has not been similarly recognized as an important aspect of understanding mental disorders; i.e., it has not informed and shaped the mainstream scientific and clinical frameworks in psychiatry. Recall that cognitive science, especially after the "cognitive revolution," was not considered a possible epistemic resource to understand psychopathology. Nor do medical students and clinical trainees receive dedicated courses and training in the human sciences. The use of *MuSe* in conjunction with the trilateral strategy enables access to the underutilized knowledge derived from human sciences.

Next, consider the clinical knowledge grounded on medicine-adjacent care disciplines, such as social work, clinical psychology, nursing, etc., as well as the clinical know-how of practicing clinicians. These clinicians have direct encounters with patients and have developed a repository of practical knowledge of the treatments and strategies that work. Some of them produce knowledge in the forms of publishing case studies, etc. Yet their knowledge has been underappreciated by the official scientific frameworks. The use of *MuSe* in conjunction with the trilateral strategy enables access to the underutilized knowledge accumulated by these care disciplines.

Finally, consider philosophy. Recall that philosophical approaches to the self played an important role in the construction of *MuSe*. By engaging with *MuSe*, psychiatry would be able to benefit from philosophy's wealth of conceptual and practical tools to think about the self and connected issues surrounding autonomy, agency and flourishing.

6.3 *MuSe* and flourishing

MuSe, in conjunction with the trilateral strategy, can enable psychiatry realize its goal to help individuals flourish by providing individuals with clinical and reflective resources to respond to mental distresses and disorders. From a clinical standpoint, the use of *MuSe* and the trilateral strategy will help clinicians develop personalized and effective tools to address an individual's mental distress. From an individual's reflective standpoint, *MuSe* will help them to think about their mental distress or disorder in a way that engages with the multiple facets of the self and allow them to develop personal strategies to strengthen their agency and autonomy. *MuSe* empowers clinicians by getting them to focus on self-related aspects of their patients' distress and use them together with the trilateral strategy, and it empowers patients by allowing them to actively participate in their recovery and flourishing—and these are not mutually exclusive.

To explain how this works, let's consider the experiences of a student, call her Janie,[1] who is shy and introverted and is usually by herself at school. Her family has few resources, and she has lost siblings to various tragedies: one struggled with epilepsy which culminated in death, and two drowned in the lake near their house. She feels she has to work hard at school to prove herself to her teachers and family, and this causes distress. She is always worried: about school, about her parents' finances, about fitting in, about her clothes, about losing another sibling to death. Janie finds refuge in writing. The only thing she wants for herself is to become a writer.

She decides that being a teacher might help her get a stable job so she can support her family and also continue writing. One day when she is doing a teaching practicum at a teachers' college, she is so nervous about being observed and graded based on her performance that she runs away; she has a meltdown in her dorm, leading her roommates to call emergency, and she ends up being hospitalized.

You are a clinician seeing Janie, trying to make sense of her distress and help her. As a first step, you take *MuSe* as your framework for interviewing her. You ask Janie to describe her physical experiences surrounding her distress; for example, whether she sweats or has heart palpitations, how her sleep has been lately, etc. You then move to her social relationships. Does she have siblings? What do her parents do? Why did being observed by her teacher cause stress? You are trying to get a picture of her relationships and her behavior in social situations. Next, you move to the experiential facet and ask Janie to say more about the recent experiences that resulted in her hospitalization. What led her to run away from the class? Why couldn't she stop crying? How did it feel to panic when she saw the teacher? Then, you dive into her overall conception of herself. Does she feel she can be a good teacher? Does she feel confident in her ability to educate children? If not, what is she worried about? Finally, you ask Janie to narrate how she views her life, her hopes and dreams and fears, and so on.

Janie responds to these questions. She tells you that she sleeps four to five hours a day, and she wants to be a teacher, but she is worried about her performance in class. If she cannot pass, she won't be able to get her certificate. She says this is important because she needs the income to support her family. She also tells you about her dreams of being a writer. You have a broad idea of what might be happening with Janie, with all the loss, grief, ongoing life stressors and pressures, but you are not sure if you should diagnose her with a form of mental disorder.

You use the trilateral strategy and recall what you have learned from psychology and cognitive science about the experience of loss during childhood. You wonder about her parents and their living conditions, and you ask for help from a social worker at the hospital to dig deeper to get a sense of the family's socioeconomic status. You recall what you learned in your cognitive science class about the factors involved in forming self-concepts and think supportive counselling may help her develop positive self-concepts. Based on your previous experience with similar patients, your knowledge of how individuals respond to life stressors, and your training in psychopharmacology, you might also recommend a low dose of antidepressant to take the edge off Janie's distress, address her sleep problems for now, and help her develop better coping skills. You record in Janie's chart that she might benefit from an anxiety disorder diagnosis so that she gains access to clinical resources. In communicating your observations and recommendations to Janie, you explain to her that there are various legitimate reasons for her to feel distressed and highlight to her that it is OK to feel overwhelmed under these circumstances. You explain to her that she might benefit from receiving an anxiety disorder diagnosis as you think her experiences can be best characterized under this label based on existing scientific and clinical knowledge and what she describes. But you also tell her that research on anxiety disorders is ongoing, and she should not think of this condition as a permanent impediment that will affect her for the rest of her life, or that she can never have a fulfilling life with anxiety present. You explain that based on what is known so far, individuals with similar experiences can respond very well to a number of interventions, including medications, social support, and a mix of self-care and management strategies, ranging from meditation to exercise, healthy diet and sleep habits, etc. You prescribe an antidepressant, refer her to the social worker who can provide supportive psychotherapy, and ask her to come and see you again in four weeks. You also say your office can help her explore resources that might help her and her family. You then point out some educational resources that can help her understand why she feels the way she does and learn from others who may have had similar experiences. Finally, you explain to her that she should not focus too much on the diagnostic label, as labels are primarily starting points for clinicians so they can ensure patients get the help they need. Instead, she should focus on cultivating reflective and somatic habits that support her mental well-being so she can continue to pursue her goals. You encourage her to continue to continue to stay vigilant about her anxiety and track if her treatment plan is helping, while continuing to pursue the activities she enjoys, like writing. You recommend some resources to deal with her heart palpitations, including the development of skills to address her panic in high-stress situations. By turning first to *MuSe* and then to the trilateral strategy, you have been able explore various intervention methods to help Janie develop better coping skills and strengthen her agency and autonomy. Ultimately, she will have access to a variety of medical and non-medical resources to respond to her distress.

Beyond assisting clinicians, *MuSe* offers helpful reflective resources for the individual with mental distress. As discussed before, individuals create self-narratives in an effort to represent and make sense of the states of affairs in their lives. They not only help individuals sort out what is happening in their lives in an orderly and manageable manner; they also guide their actions and decisions. In that sense, self-narratives are edifying: they can lead individuals to develop more or less resourceful ways to respond to the states of affairs in their lives, including the states of affairs surrounding their distresses and disorders.

The overriding need in creating a self-narrative is to make sense of what is going on in one's life. As I have pointed out, some self-narratives surrounding mental distresses and disorders are developed using a medical stance: the individual explains the current state of affairs surrounding their distress by using a medical perspective and language. Stephanie Foo, as cited in Chapter 3 is a good example; in her self-narrative, she says *everything* in her life, including her career choice and her relationships, has been shaped by her complex post-traumatic stress disorder (PTSD). Other self-narratives about mental distresses and disorders highlight and emphasize social relationships, including the individual's upbringing, family life, social role as a mother, and so on. These self-narratives draw on the properties and frameworks of the subject's social and cultural world.

Using *MuSe* might help subjects understand their experience of mental distress by situating it within the model's five facets, instead of considering mental distress or disorder as something external to self-experience. Returning to Janie, if she uses *MuSe* to reflect on her experiences as an individual, she might be encouraged to look more closely at her physical habits, such as food and exercise, to track how self-care habits intersect with her feelings of extreme worry. Similarly, she might be encouraged to reassess her worries about her parents' finances by recognizing the influence of her socioeconomic status on her life experiences and realizing that she does not have a lot of control over that. Or she might be encouraged to reach out to the resources provided by the social worker at the doctor's office. Realizing her heightened stress around others, she might decide to work on skills and strategies to reduce anxiety around others and learn to manage social situations better. She might realize that in contexts where she has low self-esteem, she tends to get nervous, so she decides to prepare more before she teaches so that she can be more confident in front of others and not panic while teaching. Most importantly, she can examine her self-narratives and contemplate developing a self-narrative which may help her cope with the challenges associated with her distress. Instead of thinking about herself through the diagnostic label of anxiety disorder, for example, she can develop a self-narrative that engages deeply with each facet of the self. If she takes a multi-faceted approach to understanding her mental distress, she may develop the capacity to strengthen her agency and autonomy by working on each facet. She may discover that her self-narrative about wanting to be a writer is powerful and use that knowledge to guide future decisions, from reorganizing her day so that she makes time for writing to choosing a university that may help her realize her goals.

Note that in a multifaceted approach to understanding mental distress, a different facet may be more important for each individual. For some, physical self-concepts may be more salient: if a former top athlete becomes disabled during war and has PTSD-like experiences, part of their response to PTSD could be doing more work to develop a self-narrative that strengthens their self-concept, i.e., a self-narrative that is not primarily focused on physical ability.

Work in cognitive science supports the claim that if the subject is able to connect their mental distress to their specific life experiences, they will develop adaptive cognitive responses. For example, some psychologists contend that when individuals write about traumatic experiences by deeply engaging with the associated emotional difficulties in their lives, significant physical and mental health follows (Pennebaker 1997). This is referred to as the "disclosure phenomenon." Furthermore, talking and writing about emotional experiences yields comparably higher biological, mood, and cognitive effects than talking or writing about superficial topics (Pennebaker 1997). While some of the positive outcomes of the disclosure phenomenon are due to a reduction in inhibition, many researchers argue the basic cognitive and linguistic processes involved in writing are more significant factors. There is a connection between language and health outcomes (Pennebaker 1993). More thoughtful writing, it is suggested, leads to better health outcomes, as does the use of positive emotion words. Similar forces might be at play in grief-related distress. Perhaps stripping away these self- or context-related aspects of the encounter with mental disorder may prevent a patient's concerns from being effectively addressed in treatment contexts (Sadler 2005; Tekin 2015).

6.4 MuSe and science: expertise and objectivity

MuSe, in conjunction with the trilateral strategy, also helps psychiatry meet its commitment to scientific objectivity by turning psychiatry's attention to previously underutilized epistemic resources and offering more nuanced and sophisticated notions of expertise and objectivity. Recall that one of the fundamental reasons for psychiatry to stay away from concepts like the self or subjectivity is what I termed the *Freud problem* in Chapter 2, i.e., the assumption that the self is a psychoanalytic concept, and its use will make it impossible for psychiatry to establish scientific objectivity. In addition, as I explained in Chapter 2, the request to include patients in the scientific decision-making process during the DSM-5 revisions was denied on the grounds that it would spoil scientific objectivity.

I take the objectivity challenge head on here. The self can be studied objectively, and patients can be included in knowledge production—the real problem is the meaning of scientific objectivity. Simply stated, psychiatry needs to adjust its approach to scientific objectivity by applying more sophisticated notions of expertise and objectivity. In particular, mobilizing *MuSe* and the trilateral strategy, I underscore that self-reports of individuals diagnosed with mental disorders are indispensable to our understanding of mental disorder. These self-reports are an integral part of the picture of the individual drawn using *MuSe*, and they build up the testimonial knowledge that serves as the third aspect of the trilateral strategy. In addition, as I argued in the previous chapter, at least some patients can be considered experience-based experts, and their direct contribution to epistemic practices in psychiatry, such as participating on committees making decisions about psychiatric categories and classifications, provides unmatched resources.

Recognizing the value of self-reports and thinking of at least some patients as experts by experience underscore that knowledge is situated, and the social location of agents enhances or limits what they know (Wylie 2015). In this sense, patients have tacit and experiential knowledge and expertise that is not shared by clinicians or psychiatrists. Their mental disorders and their diagnoses shape the material conditions of their lives and the conceptual resources through which they represent and interpret these experiences. Their self-reports give us access to their orientational challenges, their social and cultural contexts, and the conditions that enabled them to cope with their experiences and find their niche. All these insights allow clinicians to contemplate which ways of labeling or framing these experiences will be most conducive to flourishing. In addition, although the dominant view assumes otherwise, patients' direct involvement in knowledge-building practices in psychiatry does not spoil scientific objectivity. Quite the opposite, in fact: inclusion of individuals who have experience-based expertise on mental disorders in scientific decision-making enhances scientific objectivity.

Let's revisit the controversy around including patients in the DSM-5 revision process and see how the more sophisticated notions of expertise and objectivity emphasized by *MuSe* and the trilateral strategy serve psychiatry's scientific commitments. Recall from Chapter 2 that historically, the DSM was developed and revised mostly by psychiatrists who were members of the American Psychiatric Association, albeit representing different backgrounds and research areas in psychiatry. In the DSM-I, the Veterans Administration was also involved in the decision-making process as the decisions were pivotal for determining who was fit to serve in the military. Starting with the DSM-III, there was an effort to diversify the DSM task force membership to include researchers with different interests and a wider spectrum of psychiatrists, for example, women. Thus, the DSM creation and revision process has always been a collaborative epistemic ritual (Solomon 2015) involving a community of researchers and clinicians from different working groups studying different mental disorders.

Prior to the publication of the DSM-5, various groups, including patients, caregivers, mental health activists, advocacy groups, philosophers, and clinicians, invited the APA to involve patients in the revision process by including them on the DSM-5 task force or in a working group. As discussed in Chapter 2, some invoked social and political reasons by highlighting the need for the process to be democratic and to include all stakeholders, i.e., members of the public with a direct interest in the diagnostic criteria, such as patients and their families (Sadler and Fulford 2004). Others approached it from the perspective of patient advocacy and emphasized the need "for scientific experts to review their nosological recommendations in light of rigorous consideration of consumer experience and feedback" (Stein and Phillips 2013). Some clinicians cited epistemic reasons and argued patients bring a different perspective to the conversation on psychiatric classifications because they can report on their subjective experiences, and such reports can enable mental health professionals to be more empathetic (Flanagan, Davidson, and Strauss 2010).

The DSM-5 task force initially appeared sympathetic to the social and political reasons, as it acknowledged the potential benefits of patients' inclusion, given the collaborative nature of DSM construction. However, it suggested the time prior to publication was too limited for an elaborate engagement. It suggested the APA's call for feedback from the public through an online forum on DSM-5 was a positive step towards including patient input, insofar as patients are also members of the general public.

The DSM-5 task force's response was problematic in that patients' potential contributions were framed as having the same value as those of the general public—the ability of their unique standpoint, as those directly encountering mental disorder, to improve the diagnostic criteria for mental disorders was dismissed. The notion of expertise was limited to those with training in medicine and psychiatry, and patients were not considered experts. The task force's argument against patient inclusion was that the "subjectivity of the data" in patients' reports conflicted with psychiatry's desire to establish itself as an objective form of inquiry (Regier et al. 2010). In the end, the DSM-5 was published without patient input, either on the task force or in the working groups. Ironically, the publication of the DSM-5 was delayed another three years after all these conversations, and this was arguably enough time to include patients in the process. Yet it did not happen. So it is hard to take seriously the reasoning that there was not enough time. Simply stated, patients were not invited to provide systematic feedback by virtue of their status as patients.

More importantly, if psychiatry is guided by the *MuSe* framework and the trilateral strategy, patient inclusion does not damage psychiatry's goal to achieve scientific objectivity; rather, it enhances it. Let's turn to the task force's worries and see how these can be addressed by the *MuSe* framework and the trilateral strategy. The worries were stated as the following:

> We recognize that subjecting criteria to patient review may allow DSM-V to draw a more complete and clinically meaningful picture of disorders based on individual experiences … of patients. … Integrating objective diagnostic criteria and patient-subjective data may serve to enhance the therapeutic alliance, since it could assist the clinician in better understanding the source of an individual patient's distress, not simply the clinician's preconceived assertions about what a given diagnosis is and is not. By definition, subjectivity is variable from person to person, therefore making it impossible to develop definitive criteria that would apply to every disorder.
>
> (Regier et al. 2010, 308)

As philosopher Heather Douglas rightly points out, there are different senses of objectivity in science, and they are all important and valid (Douglas 2000). The key to doing science and achieving objectivity is to determine what sense of objectivity is a better fit for the scientific practice in question. In the preceding citation from Regier et al. (2010), the task force does not define precisely what it means by "objective" or "subjective" in the context of the DSM revisions. Appealing to contemporary philosophers of science, I unpack the three assumptions the DSM creators make about objectivity (Douglas 2004; Longino 1990). These assumptions are remnants of two logical positivistic views of what science is: 1) objectivity as the opposite of subjectivity; and 2) objectivity as concordance. Both are reminiscent of the logical positivistic notion of objectivity, and neither fits the purposes of inquiry in psychiatry.

According to logical positivism, knowledge is based on either logical reasoning or empirical experience. When the objectivity of scientific knowledge is evaluated, the focus is on the outcome of scientific inquiry. Justifiable evidence constitutes observational data, enabled when scientists apply a "view from nowhere" perspective to the phenomenon under investigation. The detachment reflects the value neutrality of scientific knowledge. Thus, in this view, science is objective to the extent to which it is detached from researchers' perspectives and values, and evidence is grounded on impartial (third-person) observational data verified by the world. Otherwise stated, objective science is impartial, value-neutral, and uncontestable.

One of the methods of scientific inquiry adopted by logical positivists to attain this goal is operationalism. Operational definitions characterize an otherwise complex scientific phenomenon by defining its features in a way that easily lends itself to scientific measurement and analysis. As discussed in Chapter 2, operationalism was adopted in the DSM formulation, starting with DSM-III, with observable signs and symptoms becoming the defining features of mental disorders.

In the DSM-5 task force's statement above, the first assumption is 1) objectivity is the opposite of subjectivity (Regier et al. 2010). In the citation, "objective diagnostic criteria" and "patient-subjective data" are juxtaposed. Their relationship is framed as complementary; working together, they "serve to enhance the therapeutic alliance" and "assist the clinician in better understanding the source of an individual patient's distress" (Regier et al. 2010). Although not explained, "objective diagnostic criteria" seem to refer to the symptoms (observed by the patient) and signs (observed by others) of mental disorders, as starting with DSM-III, symptoms and signs were considered observable features of mental disorders, with the same phenomenon consistently appearing across different settings. What seems to be the main difference between "objective diagnostic criteria" and "patient-subjective data," then, is whether the encounter with mental distress is reported from the third-person perspective or the first-person perspective. "Patient-subjective data" seem to be patients' self- reports about their experiences, and "objective diagnostic criteria" seem to be third-person reports, presumably observable by clinicians.

The conception of objectivity as the opposite of subjectivity is reminiscent of the positivistic view that science is only objective if its observations and theories reflect a view from nowhere, independent of scientists' subjective perspectives. Thinking of objectivity as the opposite of subjectivity is a limited interpretation of complex concepts used in myriad ways in scientific practices and philosophy of science (Douglas 2004). Douglas argues conceiving objectivity as the opposite of subjectivity represents a kind of "detached objectivity," with an attempt to maintain a metaphorical "distance" or "detachment" between "the knower and the subject" (Douglas 2004). Such detachment or distance is thought to keep the individual observer from being overly invested in a particular outcome or fearing another, thus biasing/spoiling their understanding of the phenomenon in question. In the positivistic view, science should be based on impartial or third-person observations, not "subjective" or first-person perspectives.

In the above statement, when the DSM-5 task force raises questions about using "patient-subjective data" by citing variability from person to person, it seems to want diagnostic criteria to be "detached" and "impartial," with a distance between the knower and the subject. Such impartiality or detachment is assumed to be only possible through the third-person observations of clinicians, hence the preference for "objective diagnostic criteria." Patients' self-reports are framed as obstacles to achieving this kind of objectivity.

However, this does not fit the goals of inquiry in psychiatry. The subject matter of psychiatry is mental disorder, a phenomenon that directly affects the individual in question. Patients' self-reports and their expertise on their own experiences are not only constitutive of mental disorders but are also epistemically indispensable to identify the properties of mental disorders and subsequently develop treatments—the main goal of psychiatry as a scientific and medical discipline. In fact, the research generated by the working groups in the DSM revision process includes knowledge generated by clinicians from their encounter with patients. In other words, the DSM is not against including knowledge about patient subjectivity in knowledge-building practices but is against directly involving patients as subjects of knowledge and builders of knowledge, rather than objects of inquiry studied by clinicians.

Thus, the assumption that objectivity is the opposite of subjectivity is invalid; it is not the right type of objectivity for psychiatry, even though it can be a useful characterization of objectivity in the context of another kind of science. We have to understand what each subject is experiencing to determine if their experience is a typical feature of the mental disorder in question. The knowledge offered by subjective reports cannot be construed as ancillary to the knowledge possessed by medical professionals; rather, these subjective standpoints are necessary for a fine-grained, objective understanding of mental disorders. As discussed in the previous chapter, self-reports provide rich information on the encounter with mental disorder that is not immediately available to clinicians. In short, subjectivity and objectivity in the context of psychiatric knowledge are not opposites; the former is necessary for the latter. We must strive for a pluralism that combines patients' perspectives with those of medical professionals and researchers to acquire knowledge in psychiatry.

The second assumption made by the DSM-5 task force is the construal of 2) objectivity as concordance. As seen in the DSM creation and revision processes, the goal is to reach agreement between trained experts. When the DSM-5 task force expresses worry about patient involvement, it questions "whose subjective point of view is to be considered." If more than one patient is reporting on experiences of illness or the social context, whose experience must be taken as representative? Various reports on the same disorder, e.g., PTSD, may very well be contradictory. The task force's worry is that no single perspective will have the uncontested agreement of all participants. It seems concerned about how to square expert judgments with patient judgments. The DSM-5 task force is interested in attaining what Douglas calls "concordant objectivity," which requires the agreement of all involved experts with the perspective offered. Concordant objectivity leaves no room for interaction, debate, or conversation among participants. However, the DSM's revision practices themselves do not align with this assumption. There is constant critical engagement in diagnostic criteria, evident in the working groups' reports to the task force.

The DSM creation and revision process is interactive and based on collective decision-making, even though there are often disagreements between the members. For example, during the DSM-5 revisions, there was serious consideration of classifying personality disorders qualitatively, rather than quantitatively, using a dimensional approach. Personality disorders were historically conceptualized categorically: the individual was thought to either have or not have the disorder. However, based on recent research, a significant number of psychiatrists involved in the DSM-5 revisions proposed to categorize personality disorders in dimensions, according to which the symptoms would be ranked on a spectrum ranging from less to more severe. This was new because the traditional categorical classifications based on the presence or absence of symptoms did not consider the degree of severity. While initially it looked like this change was going to go through, in the end it did not: personality disorder classifications remained the same. My point is that the ideal of objectivity as concordance is not actually followed by the DSM, and the revision process includes ongoing disagreements and debates and collective decision-making. Thus, denying patient inclusion on the grounds that it would ruin the DSM's concordant objectivity is inconsistent with DSM practices.

The assumptions apparent in the task force's concerns about patient inclusion, i.e., objectivity as the opposite of subjectivity and objectivity as concordance, do not align with psychiatry's goal as a branch of medicine and science. Psychiatry's target of inquiry is mental disorder, and this is necessarily encountered by a subject. Therefore, engaging with patients' perspectives on their experiences is integral to arriving at knowledge. Patients' accounts of their encounter with mental disorder (subjective) are directly relevant for making sense of the phenomenon, thus obtaining a more accurate picture of both the nature of the mental disorder and its treatment. In addition, expecting to arrive at a concordant account, wherein the judgments of all experts in the process concur on a particular observation, is not a plausible expectation. The phenomenon under investigation is mostly unknown, rich, and complex. This requires and invites conversation, interaction, and even conflicts between those who encounter and those who treat mental disorders. In fact, the very inclusion of differently trained experts in the current DSM creation process shows the process of inquiry is interactional, collaborative, and critical, not uncontested concordance with a certain viewpoint.

In what follows, using *MuSe* and the trilateral strategy, I propose and develop Participatory Interactive Objectivity (PIO) to address the kinds of concerns raised by the DSM-5 task force, especially those that involve adjudicating multiple perspectives of patients and psychiatrists. PIO, guided by feminist epistemologists' conception of objectivity, better fits the goals of psychiatric inquiry and can establish venues within which to settle disagreements between patients and psychiatrists in the DSM deliberation process.

PIO embodies the fundamental commitments of *MuSe* and the trilateral strategy, specifically their framework for thinking about psychiatry as a form of social epistemology, i.e., a collective enterprise shaped by a variety of scientific, medical, and testimonial practices, aiming to develop knowledge on effective treatments for mental disorders. Building on feminist philosophy of science, this framework conceptualizes psychiatric science as a community activity and takes this social feature of science to be necessary for the objectivity of scientific inquiry. *MuSe* is a model of a patient, developed based on information from human sciences about the self and the self-reports of both the individual in question and other individuals who have reported similar experiences. Similarly, the trilateral strategy is a strategy to investigate mental distresses and disorders; it directs the clinician to take seriously not just scientific and clinical knowledge when engaging with the individual patient, but also testimonial knowledge. In my vision of psychiatry guided by *MuSe* and the trilateral strategy, self-reports are epistemic building blocks of psychiatric knowledge, and at least some patients are considered experts by experience whose contribution to psychiatric knowledge is indispensable, and objectivity in psychiatry can be arrived at and maintained through PIO.

PIO challenges the assumptions about DSM objectivity held by the DSM-5 task force. Following feminist philosophers of science, it takes objectivity of science to be a process rather than an outcome. It highlights the value of procedural objectivity and includes individuals with a first-person encounter with mental disorder in the community of knowers and knowledge generators in psychiatry, thus expanding the notion of expertise to include both those trained in psychopathology and those with experiential knowledge. In addition, PIO leaves behind assumptions of objectivity as the opposite of subjectivity and objectivity as concordance because neither reflects the nature of inquiry in psychiatry. Instead, PIO sees objectivity as a participatory and interactive process of negotiation. The three elements of the trilateral strategy, i.e., appealing to scientific, clinical, and testimonial knowledge, are all part of the framework for thinking about mental disorders. What can be considered most effective clinically and what is most resourceful for patients' flourishing are determined through ongoing discussion and negotiation among individuals with mental disorders, clinicians, and scientists. Let me explain how this process works.

As Helen Longino argues, science is objective to the extent that its methods, especially its criteria for assessing theories, are neither arbitrary nor subjective. To ensure objectivity in science, we must consider it a social activity organized to permit and encourage transformative criticism—criticism with the power to change the contextual values of scientists, should they be ill-founded. Longino writes:

> From a logical point of view, if scientific knowledge were to be understood as the simple sum of finished products of individual activity, then not only would there be no way to block or mitigate the influence of subjective preference but scientific knowledge itself would be a potpourri of merrily inconsistent theories. Only if the products of inquiry are understood to be formed by the kind of critical discussion that is possible among a plurality of individuals about a commonly accessible phenomenon, can we see how they count as knowledge rather than opinion.
>
> (Longino 1990)

Scientific knowledge must not be understood as the "simple sum of finished products" of individual scientists, but as the product of collaboration and critical engagement among a plurality of scientists (Longino 1990). The social nature of scientific activity leads to the mechanism of transformative criticism, i.e., a process that facilitates the adjudication of values if they jeopardize the objectivity of science. For example, peer review of scientists' work in the publication process allows a body of knowledge to be scrutinized by a group of experts. Thus, including a diversity of scientists in the knowledge production process, along with the mechanism of transformative criticism, makes procedural objectivity possible (Longino 1990).

It is plausible to respond to the argument that inclusion of patients in the DSM revision process will compromise psychiatry's goals as an objective science by evoking Longino. Patients must be included in the knowledge production process for epistemic reasons; their inclusion will not compromise psychiatry's goal to be an objective science. The subjectivity of their experience with mental disorders and their perspectives on the diagnostic criteria are assets, not impediments, in the scientific process. Their direct encounter with mental disorder is an experience mostly unknown to clinical or scientific experts, unless, of course, these experts have encountered mental disorders themselves. Including those who have encountered mental disorders will allow transformative criticism by ensuring different points of view are part of the scientific decision-making process. This, in turn, will lead to procedural objectivity, as the scientifically and clinically trained experts and the patients can critically scrutinize each other's hypotheses and evidential reasoning, thereby limiting the intrusion of individual subjective preferences into scientific knowledge. In the process, the subjective experiences of patients may create objective patterns of experiences previously missed by clinically trained experts.

A research framework for mental disorders using *MuSe* and the trilateral strategy could incorporate a community of scientists, clinicians, and patients. While this might be considered a radical idea, the existing DSM creation process is poised to accommodate such a structure. In its present form, the DSM task force is composed of psychiatrists trained in psychopathology, as well as working groups who coordinate research on mental disorders and make recommendations on diagnostic criteria to the task force. In other words, the process is designed to be collaborative and critically engaging. The argument for the inclusion of patients in the community of knowers and critical engagers is a natural extension of this process; to ensure objectivity in psychiatry, we must recognize and encourage the social process of attaining knowledge and include not only professionals with training in psychopathology but also those with first-hand experience.

Should patients' input carry the same weight as that of psychiatrists and other scientific and clinical experts? After all, in her discussion of transformative criticism, Longino says scientists are the ultimate decision-makers, even though she highlights the importance of having a diverse community of scientists representing different viewpoints. Perhaps Longino herself is reluctant to advocate for including patients in the scientific decision-making process, as they are not scientists.

While PIO departs from Longino's discussions of transformative criticism and objectivity by promoting the inclusion of patients (i.e., non-scientists) in research and decision-making, it is consistent with Longino's contextualism insofar as it promotes viewing science as practice by highlighting the importance of paying attention to the nature of the scientific practice at hand. Because the unknowns of mental disorders are still greater than the knowns, we have to commit to the practice (rather than the product) of psychiatric research as it unfolds. If we pay attention to the nature of research in psychiatry, the inclusion of patients in the community of researchers working on mental disorders is necessary for epistemic reasons. As discussed in previous chapters, psychiatry is an intervention-oriented science; its main goal is the discovery of the scientifically relevant properties of mental disorders that yield successful explanations, reliable predictions, and effective interventions. To discover and then investigate these features, it is necessary to adopt a trilateral strategy, where we examine not only the clinical and scientific work on mental disorders but also the first-person reports of those experiencing them. Taken together, these epistemic resources may help develop interventions, as they may disclose the underlying causes of mental disorder, suggest treatment, and clarify what it is like to have a mental disorder.

As discussed in Chapter 5 on self-reports, the acceptance of patient perspectives allows us to engage with different types of evidence that might be overlooked in conventional case-reporting scenarios. For example, it is important to know the nature of schizophrenia and the kind of interventions considered helpful by clinicians, but it is also important to gather data from self-reports. I thus propose to expand the community of knowers in research in psychiatry to include patients because they are experts by experience (Collins and Evans 2002).[2]

In the context of the DSM, this means refining the categories of mental disorder in light of patient input. For example, one of the symptoms of schizophrenia listed in the DSM is "affective flattening, alogia, or avolition," defined as lacking interest in social relationships (American Psychiatric Association 2013). However, patients with schizophrenia report an intense desire but perceived inability to initiate and build such relationships (Parnas and Henriksen 2014). As this example suggests, including patients in the DSM revision process would help make the disorder descriptions more representative of patients' experiences.

Now that we have established who must participate in the knowledge-generation process in psychiatry, a second question concerns what kind of objectivity psychiatry should strive for, at least in the context of the DSM, if we were to say it is not the opposite of subjectivity or a product of concordance. According to PIO, a diverse group of experts, including both patients and psychiatrists, should be members of the DSM task force and its working groups. This means they must establish a shared decision-making process through which they can deliberate each other's standpoints, perspectives, and proposals and then make decisions.

Instead of thinking of objectivity as the opposite of subjectivity and striving for a concordance of viewpoints, we must embrace group discussion, even disagreement. Participants in the DSM revision process must be invited to argue and to ferret out the sources of their disagreements. The clinically trained experts and the patients, i.e., experience-based experts, can query each other's hypotheses and evidential reasoning, but neither inter-subjective agreement nor consensus is necessary. That said, however, shared norms of agreement must be established (in advance) to determine how conflicts and disagreements will be resolved. It is beyond the scope of this book to establish what those norms may look like, but existing models of shared decision-making processes in other fields of citizen-engaged scientific practices can serve as models (e.g., Whyte 2018). For example, we must consider the values that are a part of this process, including, but not limited to, the need for both trained experts and experience-based experts to trust the other party has a meaningful epistemic contribution to make and to remain open to criticism. In the end, including patients in the DSM development process will enhance psychiatric epistemology by encouraging transformative criticism and ensuring different points of view are part of the scientific decision-making process.

6.5 *MuSe* versus the biopsychosocial model

I have explained how the use of *MuSe*, in conjunction with the trilateral strategy, is conducive to advancing psychiatry's twin commitments of patient flourishing and scientific rigor. An important unanswered question is the nature of the relationship between *MuSe* and the biopsychosocial (BPSM) model. Like the BPSM, *MuSe* is aimed at addressing the short-comings of the biomedical model and the DSM-based approach to mental disorders, but the two models have important differences.

The BPSM was proposed in 1977 by George Engel as a means to bridge the gap between psychiatric exclusionism (i.e., Szaszian views) and reductionism. At the time, psychiatry was trying to establish itself as a legitimate form of scientific inquiry by following the biomedical model of disease, just like other areas of medicine, but had become a target of criticism for construing regular problems of living as mental disorder instead of looking at the social factors that contribute to mental health. As discussed in previous chapters, the biomedical model takes a reductionist approach to mental disorders, focuses on their underlying biological factors, and treats them through medical interventions. In contrast, the BPSM sees mental disorders as emerging in a complex interplay of biological, psychological, and social factors. While the biomedical model construes disorders as isolated physical abnormalities, the BPSM views them as outcomes of the dynamic interactions among the biological, psychological, and social factors.

Engel was worried about the rising interest in the somatic markers of mental disorders, at the expense of considering psychological and social factors. In his view, the biomedical model had shortcomings when applied to mental illness, and medicine based solely on biomedical research was inadequate and impersonal. The BPSM encourages the development of interventions targeting all these factors. It is rooted in general systems theory (i.e., looking at properties on different levels of organization) and can allow inquiry on different levels without reducing higher levels to lower ones. The BPSM recognizes that patients have their own thoughts, feelings, and history (Engel 1977).

Since its appearance, Engel's BPSM has triggered debate both within medicine, psychiatry and philosophy. Some argue the BPSM is not a model because it is entirely conceptual and does not model anything (Benning 2015). As Robert Bartz points out, "BPSMs are integrated theories of disease, not models for physician-patient interactions in family practice" (1999). Niall McLaren has similarly ruled out various things the BPSM might be a model of, including disease or treatment (McLaren 1998, 2020). Others say calling BPSM a model creates confusion among researchers who want to use it in practice, because it is vague and not explanatory or predictive (Álvarez et al. 2012), but its defenders contend it can fruitfully be applied to specific stages of specific health conditions (Bolton and Gillett 2019). There have also been worries about the BPSM's description of what constitutes "biological," "psychological," and "social." Nassir Ghaemi, for example, argues the BPSM requires a narrow, simplistic notion of biology and disease (e.g., separating biology/environment) and omits the discussion of social factors or larger society beyond the doctor-patient relationship (Ghaemi 2011). Other critics suggest the BPSM does not accommodate the subjectivity of the patient. Engel's discussion covers the biological, psychological, and sociological factors that generate disorders, but it does not allow for patients' subjective perspectives along biological, psychological, and social dimensions (Benning 2015). In related criticism, some say the BPSM cannot account for non-medically explained symptoms.

Another concern is that the BPSM does not sufficiently guide practice (Benning 2015). For example, it does not make clinicians care about empathy, curiosity, trust, etc. Some empirical studies show the BPSM is not necessarily applied well; the system hierarchy in the model does not prioritize any levels, leaving clinicians without methods for determining what to focus on (McLaren 2021). In psychiatry, the BPSM is most often applied in the context of "combined treatment" (i.e., combinations of social, pharmaceutical, and psychological treatments), "reflective processes" (i.e., helping clinicians reflect on their beliefs), and "medical education" (Álvarez et al. 2012). However, critics note that at times, treatment requires linear reasoning rather than the BPSM's circular causality (Gritti 2017). Finally, some suggest the BPSM is not widely used in healthcare because of concerns about its validity (Halligan and Wade 2017); it is vaguely defined and not operationalized in behavioral terms, making it untestable (Gritti 2017).[3]

MuSe is developed in the spirit of the BPSM in that it recognizes mental disorders must be understood and addressed in relation to biological, psychological, and social factors. But it is more specific with respect to what it models: *MuSe* is a model of the person/individual who experiences distress and demands or needs attention from others, including clinicians. As dis-cussed earlier in the chapter, it aims to guide clinicians in examining indi-viduals with mental distress, as well as the individuals themselves, activating clinical and reflective resources to develop responses to their mental distress that enable flourishing. *MuSe* is committed to understanding patients' experience of mental distress, including the biological and social factors that shape the experience. In that sense, *MuSe* not only captures the subjective dimensions of mental disorder encounter but also systematizes them, thus allowing scrutiny and intervention. In addition, *MuSe* is similar to the BPSM in that it highlights the psychological factors in the development of mental disorders, but going a step further, it calls for taking seriously the research conducted on the self that is based on human sciences when assess-ing whether someone has a mental distress or disorder and determining how it can be addressed. Finally, while the BPSM has remained silent on what role the patients' testimonies can play in medical research and treat-ment, *MuSe* not only promotes but also creates a system for the inclusion of first-person reports in psychiatric epistemology and practice.

Overall, both *MuSe* and the *BPSM* can be best characterized as products of their time, as responses to the way mental disorders are investigated. The BPSM is a response to the state of affairs in psychiatry and mental disorder treatment in the 1970s; it addresses the shortcomings of the medical model and anti-psychiatry sentiments. *MuSe* is developed in a similar spirit, as a response to the DSM-style of thinking and engaging with mental disorders, helping individuals affected by mental distress and disorder get the care they need from clinicians and society at large. It offers conceptual and pragmatic tools to think about and engage with mental disorders in the 2020s and beyond.

6.6 Conclusion

This chapter argued *MuSe*, in conjunction with the trilateral strategy, can help psychiatry meet its commitments to patient flourishing and scientific rigor. Com-bining these can provide conceptual and empirical tools for both clinicians and patients to respond to mental distress and disorder and allow psychiatry to improve its relationship to science by offering more expansive and sophisticated notions of expertise and objectivity. Section 2 explained how *MuSe* can be applied by using the trilateral strategy, an integrative framework relying on patients' self-reports, scientific research, and the clinical know-how accumulated through training and experience. Section 3 explored how *MuSe* and the trilateral strategy help meet psychiatry's goal of enabling patients to flourish by enhancing their reflective capacity to respond to their mental distresses and disorders. Section 4 showed *MuSe* and the trilateral strategy can improve psychiatry's relationship with science by arguing for a more sophisticated and expansive conception of what counts as "expertise" and as "objectivity" in knowledge generation. Section 5 compared *MuSe* to the BPSM, developed as an alternative to the medical model.

Notes

1 This hypothetical scenario is created by drawing on Janet Frame's life experiences (Chapter 1) to help imagine how *MuSe* and the trilateral strategy open up more resources for the individual than the traditional medical model under which Frame was treated.

2 I will not develop this here but I think it is plausible to include philosophers of science in the knowledge generation process in psychiatry as "interactional experts" (Collins and Evans 2002), i.e., "those who have the ability to speak the language of a discipline in the absence of an ability to practice." In an important paper on the epistemic benefits of philosophers' engagement with scientific communities, Katie Plaisance argues philosophers of science are able to acquire interactional expertise in science through their interactions with scientists and fluency in the language of science (Plaisance 2020). She writes that such interactional expertise not only offers "socio-epistemic" benefits such as the opportunity to cultivate trust with scientific communities but also can improve philosophical work and facilitate the broader uptake of philosophers' ideas. Extending Plaisance's insights into psychiatry, it is plausible to argue philosophers are well-positioned to serve as interactional experts in psychiatry and build upon their conceptual resources to translate and communicate both the trained experts' insights and the patients' insights into the nature and treatment of mental disorders.

3 Not surprisingly, given the contentious context and the criticism of its efficacy, the BPSM has been modified a number of times (e.g., Hatala 2012). Some approaches extend "biopsychosocial approaches" to include subjectivity (Brenner 2016).

References

Álvarez, Ana Sabela, Marco Pagani, and Paolo Meucci. 2012. The Clinical Application of the Biopsychosocial Model in Mental Health: A Research Critique. *American Journal of Physical Medicine & Rehabilitation* 91(13), S173.

American Psychiatric Association. 2013. *Diagnostic and Statistical Manual of Mental Disorders*. 5th ed. Washington, DC: American Psychiatric Association.

Bartz, Robert. 1999. Beyond the Biopsychosocial Model New Approaches to Doctor-Patient Interactions. *Journal of Family Practice* 48, 601–607.

Benning, Tony. 2015. Limitations of the Biopsychosocial Model in Psychiatry. *Advances in Medical Education and Practice* 6, 347–352.

Bolton, Derek and Grant Gillett. 2019. *The Biopsychosocial Model of Health and Disease*. Cham: Palgrave Macmillan.

Brenner, Adam M. 2016. Revisiting the Biopsychosocial Formulation: Neuroscience, Social Science, and the Patient's Subjective Experience. *Academic Psychiatry* 40(5). doi:10.1007/s40596-016-0542-y.

Collins, H.M. and Robert Evans. 2002. "The Third Wave of Science Studies: Studies of Expertise and Experience." *Social Studies of Science* 32(2). doi:10.1177/0306312702032002003.

Douglas, Heather. 2000. Inductive Risk and Values in Science. *Philosophy of Science* 67(4), 559–579. doi:10.1086/392855.

Douglas, Heather. 2004. The Irreducible Complexity of Objectivity. *Synthese* 138(3), 453–473.

Engel, George. 1977. The Need for a New Medical Model: A Challenge for Biomedicine. *Science* 196(4286), 129–136. doi:10.1126/science.847460.

Flanagan, Elizabeth H., Larry Davidson, and John S. Strauss. 2010. The Need for Patient-Subjective Data in the DSM and the ICD. *Psychiatry: Interpersonal and Biological Processes* 73(4), 297–307. doi:10.1521/psyc.2010.73.4.297.

Ghaemi, S. Nassir. 2011. The Biopsychosocial Model in Psychiatry: A Critique. *Existenz* 6(1). https://existenz.us/volumes/Vol.6-1Ghaemi.html.

Gritti, Paolo. 2017. The Bio-Psycho-Social Model Forty Years Later: A Critical Review. *Journal of Psychosocial Systems* 1, 36–41.

Halligan, Peter and Derick Wade. 2017. The Biopsychosocial Model of Illness: A Model Whose Time has Come. *Clinical Rehabilitation* 31, 995–1004.

Hatala, Andrew R. 2012. The Status of the 'Biopsychosocial' Model in Health Psychology: Towards an Integrated Approach and a Critique of Cultural Conceptions. *Open Journal of Medical Psychology* 1(4). doi:10.4236/ojmp.2012.14009.

Longino, Helen E. 1990. *Science as Social Knowledge: Values and Objectivity in Scientific Inquiry*. Princeton, NJ: Princeton University Press.

McLaren, Niall. 1998. A Critical Review of the Biopsychosocial Model. *Australian & New Zealand Journal of Psychiatry* 32(1), 86–92.

McLaren, Niall. 2020. The Biopsychosocial Model: The End of a Reign of Error. *Ethical Human Psychology and Psychiatry* 22(2), 71–82.

Parnas, Josef and Mads Gram Henriksen. 2014. Disordered Self in the Schizophrenia Spectrum: A Clinical and Research Perspective. *Harvard Review of Psychiatry* 22 (5), 251–265. doi:10.1097/HRP.0000000000000040.

Pennebaker, James W. 1993. Putting Stress into Words: Health, Linguistic, and Therapeutic Implications. *Behaviour Research and Therapy* 31(6), 539–548. doi:10.1016/0005-7967(93)90105-4.

Pennebaker, James W. 1997. Writing about Emotional Experiences as a Therapeutic Process. *Psychological Science* 8(3), 162–166.

Plaisance, Kathryn S. 2020. The Benefits of Acquiring Interactional Expertise: Why (Some) Philosophers of Science Should Engage Scientific Communities. *Studies in History and Philosophy of Science* 83, 53–62.

Regier, Darrel A., Emily A. Kuhl, David J. Kupfer, and James P. McNulty. 2010. Patient Involvement in the Development of DSM-V. *Psychiatry: Interpersonal and Biological Processes* 73(4), 308–310. doi:10.1521/psyc.2010.73.4.308.

Sadler, John Z. 2005. *Values and Psychiatric Diagnosis*. Oxford: Oxford University Press.

Sadler, John Z. and Bill Fulford. 2004. Should Patients and Their Families Contribute to the DSM-V Process?. *Psychiatric Services* 55(2), 133–138. doi:10.1176/appi.ps.55.2.133.

Solomon, Miriam. 2015. *Making Medical Knowledge*. Oxford: Oxford University Press.

Stein, Dan J. and Katharine A. Phillips. 2013. Patient Advocacy and DSM-5. *BMC Medicine* 11(1), 133. doi:10.1186/1741-7015-11-133.

Tekin, Şerife. 2015. Against Hyponarrating Grief: Incompatible Research and Treatment Interests in the DSM-5. In *The DSM-5 in Perspective*, edited by Steeves Demazeux and Patrick Singy, pp. 179–197. Dordrecht: Springer Netherlands. doi:10.1007/978-94-017-9765-8_11.

Whyte, K. 2018. What Do Indigenous Knowledges Do for Indigenous Peoples?. In *Traditional Ecological Knowledge: Learning from Indigenous Practices for*

Environmental Sustainability, edited by M. Nelson and D. Shilling. Cambridge: Cambridge University Press.

Wylie, Alison. 2015. A Plurality of Pluralisms: Collaborative Practice in Archaeology. In *Objectivity in Science*, edited by Flavia Padovani, Alan Richardson, and Jonathan Y. Tsou, pp. 189–210. Cham: Springer International Publishing. doi:10.1007/978-3-319-14349-1_10.

Chapter 7

The Multitudinous Self Model and substance use disorders

7.1 Introduction

> Since I've been in this program I've not been in trouble with the law. No
> more in and out of jail. That cycle door has stopped! Thanks to this study, I
> have a job and my life back.
>
> (A patient in SALOME clinical trial, Supporters of Salome 2017)

My fundamental argument in the book is that mental distresses and disorders
are best construed in relation to the concept of the self. I further suggest the
Multitudinous Self Model (*MuSe*) is a useful instrument to meet psychiatry's
scientific and clinical commitments and enable the flourishing of individuals
with mental distresses and disorders. In this chapter, I apply the five fundamental facets of *MuSe* (i.e., physical, social, experiential, conceptual, and
narrative) and the trilateral strategy (i.e., the use of testimonial, scientific, and
clinical knowledge) to engage with substance use disorders (SUDs), which are
broadly associated with continued use of drugs despite their negative consequences for the individual. Consistent with the distinction I made between
mental distress and disorder in Chapter 5, I take SUDs to be types of mental
distress surrounding drug use that are managed in the medical system. I do
not provide a description of SUDs in a metaphysical sense with necessary and
sufficient conditions; rather, I use the label of SUD pragmatically and circumstantially, reserving its use to individuate instances of mental distress that
are examined and treated in medical contexts in health management systems.
To be considered to have an SUD, an individual must receive a medical
diagnosis or treatment or must identify themselves as having an SUD by
adopting a medical stance to make sense of their experiences, i.e., interpreting
their experiences through the language of medicine.

SUDs are diagnosed using the criteria listed in the DSM-5, for reasons
discussed in previous chapters. Interventions include a combination of
detoxification, cognitive and behavioral therapies, medication-assisted
therapies in a variety of settings such as outpatient counseling, intensive
outpatient treatment, inpatient treatment, and long-term therapeutic

DOI: 10.4324/9781003055556-10

communities, such as sober living communities. In addition, clinicians often encourage patients with SUD diagnoses to seek out and participate in non-medical communities such as Alcoholics Anonymous (AA) to create an accountability and support network.

A popular approach to understanding the causal mechanisms underlying SUD is the brain disease model, according to which SUD is a "chronic and relapsing brain disease that results from the prolonged effects of drugs on the brain" (Leshner 1997, 45). Simply stated, SUD is considered a consequence of fundamental changes in the brain's reward mechanism, generated by substance use. In the brain disease model, the elucidation of the biological mechanisms underlying SUD is seen as the key to the development of effective treatments, such as anti-addiction medications. Available treatment strategies subscribe to the brain disease model to varying degrees when it comes to treating individuals in a non-stigmatizing way. The model suggests that an individual with SUD has a disease and is not simply weak-willed. Significant resources are devoted to investigating the brain mechanisms involved in SUD, and many believe this will *eventually* lead to the development of effective interventions. The brain disease model paradigm is prevalent in research programs, such as the National Institute of Mental Health's (NIMH) Research Domain Criteria (RDoC) project, which sets "positive valence systems (reward learning, reward valuation)" as a fundamental target of its research matrix and supports relevant research in animal and human models (Kozak and Cuthbert 2016).

My goal in this chapter is to show *MuSe*, in conjunction with the tri-lateral strategy, provides more resources for flourishing than the brain disease model, both clinically and personally. That is not to say the brain disease model is wrong or research on the brain's reward systems must stop; rather, *MuSe* provides immediately available resources to enhance both clinical and scientific work on SUDs. Owing to its limited scope, the brain disease model loses sight of the individual, social, and cultural complexity of the experiences of those with substance use problems. While this model can be instrumental in unpacking some of the microcellular mechanisms involved in how substances interact with the brain's reward system, it alone cannot aid individuals' flourishing, at least not at this point in the scientific research.

Section 2 examines how the brain disease model of SUDs engages with individuals with substance use problems. Section 3 juxtaposes *MuSe*-based engagement with an individual with an SUD diagnosis to the brain disease model, highlighting how the former offers comparatively more clinical and reflective resources. Section 4 gives an overview of a study evaluating the explanatory power of *MuSe* in understanding SUDs among veterans. Section 5 zooms into substitution therapy, a controversial method to address opioid use disorder (OUD), and argues this form of treatment is successful because it demonstrates a deep engagement with the fundamental aspects of *MuSe* and adopts a trilateral strategy, bringing together testimonial, scientific, and clinical knowledge. Overall, the chapter illustrates the main argument of the book: *MuSe* promotes the development of strategies that enable flourishing while simultaneously enhancing scientific practices in psychiatry.

7.2 The brain disease model and the individual

SUD is characterized as involving a powerful and repeated motivation to consume a substance for its short-term rewards, despite the knowledge of its long-term negative consequences (West and Brown 2013, 18). The DSM-5-TR defines SUD as a problematic pattern of using a substance that results in impairment in daily life or causes noticeable distress (American Psychiatric Association 2022). For a person to be diagnosed with SUD, they must display two of 11 symptoms within the past 12 months: 1) consuming more substance than planned; 2) worrying about stopping or consistently failing efforts to control use; 3) spending a large amount of time using a substance or doing whatever is needed to obtain it; 4) failing to fulfill major obligations at home or work because of substance use; 5) "craving" the substance; 6) continuing the use of a substance despite health problems caused or worsened by it; 7) continuing the use of a substance despite its negative effects on relationships with others; 8) repeatedly using the substance in dangerous situations; 9) giving up or reducing activities because of substance use; 10) building up a tolerance to the substance; and 11) experiencing withdrawal symptoms, such as anxiety, irritability, fatigue, nausea, vomiting, hand tremors or seizures, after stopping use.

The DSM is silent on the etiology of SUD, but the brain disease model links SUD to fundamental changes in the brain's mechanisms generated by such substances as alcohol or opioids. The model restricts itself to the biological mechanisms underlying SUD and delineates the addictive process in the following way. Certain substances such as alcohol or opioids are hypothesized to directly or indirectly affect dopamine signaling in the mesolimbocortical pathway. Dopamine, colloquially known as the "feel-good neurotransmitter," is largely responsible for regulating the way individuals feel pleasure and satisfaction from activities such as eating, engaging in social interaction, or having sex. The mesolimbocortical circuit is a pathway in the brain that is individuated at both structural and functional levels. With respect to brain structure, it connects the limbic system—the mechanism processing emotions and memory—to the orbitofrontal cortex of the brain, an area involved in the cognitive process of decision-making (Hyman 1996, 2007; Ortiz et al. 1995). With respect to function, it is involved in decision-making based on the emotions generated in response to external reward stimuli. In short, it is associated with reward, appetitive motivation, and hedonic processes (Salamone and Correa 2012; Salamone et al. 2005; Schultz 2016).

Research on the precise mechanism of the brain's reward system is not conclusive. Some argue this mechanism illuminates "the profound disruptions in decision-making ability and emotional balance displayed by persons with drug addiction" (Volkow et al. 2016, 364). The predominant view is that the interaction between substances such as alcohol and the mesolimbocortical pathway produces substance use-related behaviors (Volkow et al. 2016). When individuals engage in social interactions or eating, dopamine is released to signal reward from the pleasurable activity. This encourages the individual to seek similar rewards by repeating the activity. According to the brain disease model, substances of abuse disrupt the mechanism of the mesolimbocortical pathway because they cause sharp increases in dopamine release; these, in turn, "elicit a reward signal that triggers associative learning or conditioning," and the "repeated experiences of reward become associated with the environmental stimuli that precede them" (Volkow et al. 2016, 364). This purportedly explains why and how individuals associate certain stimuli (e.g., the environment of drug-taking, persons with whom drugs are consumed, etc.) with the drug use and the pleasure associated therewith. Environmental cues may trigger the craving for and use of substances. Such conditioned responses become deeply ingrained, often lasting long after active drug use has ceased (Volkow et al. 2016, 366).

One consequence of repeated consumption of substances, according to the brain disease model, is the "desensitization of reward circuits," dampening the ability to derive pleasure from everyday activities (Volkow et al. 2016, 363). Other, more "ordinary, healthful rewards," such as eating or social interactions, "lose their former motivational power," and individuals crave drugs to achieve the same pleasure and satisfaction levels (Volkow et al. 2016, 366). In this process, executive cognition processes, such as "capacities for self-regulation [and] decision making" are impaired, leading the individual to search for "the more potent release of dopamine produced by the drug and its cues" and weakening the ability "to resist strong urges or to follow through on decisions to stop taking the drug" (Volkow et al. 2016, 366, 367).

The brain disease model of addiction is pervasive in the medical and scientific communities, as it is considered to be the key to removing the stigma of addiction (Leshner 1997; Volkow 2018; Volkow et al. 2016). The model offers important insights into SUD's physical dimensions, and the underlying biology might explain how an SUD progresses over time. However, it is limited in that the scientific evidence on the accuracy of the framework is inconclusive, and the model has not yet led to a clear set of practical and effective interventions. Some significant research has appeared within the context of NIMH's RDoC. As discussed in Chapter 2, NIMH's RDoC comprise five research domains: negative valence systems (fear, anxiety, loss); positive valence systems (reward learning, reward valuation); cognitive systems (attention, perception, working memory, cognitive control); systems for social processes (attachment formation, social communication, perception of self, perception of others); arousal/modulatory systems (arousal, circadian rhythm, sleep and wakefulness) (Kozak and Cuthbert 2016, 289). The positive valence system domain for reward circuitry is of special interest to researchers who study SUD. Ongoing research is attempting to use the RDoC framework to connect the neurobiological mechanisms involved in the brain's reward system to behavioral domains to develop preventative interventions. The thinking is that distinct neurocognitive trajectories recognized as precursors or risk factors for SUD can be targeted, engaged, and modified for addiction prevention (Rezapour et al. 2024).

Important concerns about the brain disease model have been raised by researchers, clinicians, and philosophers. Some fear it is deterministic and does not account for the individual's social and contextual differences in recovery and remission, while others suggest it generates feelings of helplessness and does not empower individuals (see Heather et al. 2022; Pickard and Ahmed 2018). I will not discuss these criticisms in detail here. My main concern with the brain disease model in the context of this chapter is its limited applicability in clinical contexts. As I observed earlier in the book, there is a disconnect between psychiatry's scientific aspirations and research programs and its immediate clinical needs, with the latter often guided in a haphazard way without a unifying clinical framework to approach individuals with mental distresses and disorders. This problem presents itself in the context of SUD; not many frameworks for intervention bridge the scientific and clinical aspects of SUD. Specifically, while extensive basic science research is being conducted using the brain disease model with the hope of developing effective interventions sometime in the future, the model does not offer resourceful pathways for individuals struggling with SUD in the present; research on applied clinical frameworks is not prominent. Kathryn Tabb astutely identifies this as a "diachronic distributive justice," or simply a "diachronic justice" problem (Tabb 2017). In Tabb's view, diachronic justice is the equitable distribution of resources between the populations of the same interest groups at two or more different times. The two interest groups affected by RDoC research on the brain disease model are individuals needing effective treatments now and individuals who will need effective treatments in the future. Given its almost exclusive focus on the biomarkers of mental disorders and the redirection of resources away from clinical research in fields such as epidemiology and psychopharmacology towards the basic sciences like genetics, biochemistry, and especially neuroscience, RDoC, in practice, assumes the long-term benefits of basic science research are more important than the short-term goals of clinical research "insofar as basic science can be expected to revolutionize patient care for countless future generations." (Tabb 2017, 1; Tabb 2020). Unfortunately, Tabb notes, the search for the biomarkers of mental disorders has not translated into significant clinical advances and has put long-term gains first, at the expense of more immediate gains, such as connecting biological processes to the human environments, social factors, and behaviors that shape and define mental disorders (Tabb 2023).

Because the brain disease model does not have a clear picture of the individual who is subject to SUD—other than a generic person with a faulty brain reward system—it does not engage with the individual's self-related characteristics and capacities, including sociality, reflectivity, decision-making, and reasoning, which, as first-person reports demonstrate, enable individuals to participate actively in their recovery and flourishing. In addition, as Hanna Pickard highlights in her work on the self, identity, and substance use, drug use for some individuals fulfills a purpose; it offers forms of positive self-identity and social experience, which they might otherwise lack, and engaging with the meaning of drug use for the user is crucial in addressing their concerns (Pickard 2021). All these considered, *MuSe* offers a helpful clinical and personal framework for thinking about SUDs for those affected by them at the moment.

7.3 *MuSe* and the individual

MuSe, in conjunction with the trilateral strategy, provides a helpful strategy to approach the individual experiencing an SUD. If used by clinicians and the individual themselves, it can help individuals develop capacities that enable their flourishing. In what follows, I examine an individual's experience with SUD using *MuSe* and explain how to develop treatment using the trilateral strategy. Engaging with an individual's experience in a way that prioritizes how the individual views their substance use patterns through the physical, social, experiential, conceptual, and narrative facets of *MuSe* and then exposing this experience to existing knowledge on how SUD can be managed may suggest multiple avenues for intervention by both clinicians and individuals with SUD, facilitating the individual's development of cognitive capacities to strengthen autonomy and agency.

MuSe construes SUD to be a person-level phenomenon, and its five facets can be used to build an empirically responsive picture of the individual, in contrast to the brain disease model, whose primary unit of analysis is the brain. Brain mechanisms are part of the picture of SUD in *MuSe*, in so far as they are part of the physical facet of the model, with direct impacts on the remaining four facets, but they are not the exclusive target. In the spirit of the instrumental use of psychiatric labels such as SUD, when the individual first arrives at the clinic, it is best to approach them as an individual with distressing substance use patterns, not as an emblem of all persons with SUD. Here, the five facets of *MuSe* are particularly helpful.

The features of the individual with problematic substance use patterns can be examined through the *physical facet* of *MuSe*. These include the central nervous system, the brain's reward system, hormones, genes, and existing disorders, such as chronic pain, diabetes, and so on. Information about the physical facets gleaned from scientific, clinical, and testimonial contexts can be used to create screening questions to gather pertinent information in the clinic. It is important, for instance, for the clinician to ask the individual presenting at the clinic if they have existing disorders, such as chronic back pain, as these may have been involved in the decision to start using substances in the first place, perhaps to alleviate the pain.

Moreover, the physical effects of drugs like alcohol or opioids can be examined using the trilateral strategy, i.e., drawing on testimonial, scientific, and clinical knowledge. A familiar clinical story is that the individual was initially attracted to the pleasant physical sensations and relaxation associated with consumption. For example, alcohol may help the individual fall asleep, or opioids might lighten physical pain. Dependency develops gradually, through the incremental increase in the consumption of the drug over time, coupled with an increased toleration of its effects. Ultimately, the individual is in a situation where they are unable to control their substance use despite feeling its negative effects. Most scientific research using the brain disease model is geared towards understanding the reward mechanisms involved. First-person reports can shed light on these mechanisms. For example, Ivana Grahovac reports her opioid dependence developed because of an unaddressed eating disorder. She says she "sought solace in substances while suffering from the illness" and eventually turned to heroin after trying it socially (Holpuch 2017). After a while, she started "needing" heroin for survival and experienced withdrawal symptoms when opioids were not available. The physical dependency led her to try everything she could to obtain opioids, including stealing money and engaging in sex work. One winter, she ended up living on the streets of Detroit. She was found in jail by a private investigator hired by her parents, where she was serving a 54-day sentence for stealing a car. She went in and out of short-term addiction treatment facilities six times but failed to get on a stable path to recovery.

If the clinician had engaged Ivana by asking about the physical facet of her self experience, the relationship between the physical aspects of the substance use patterns and the other facets of *MuSe* might have become apparent. In fact, one advantage of using *MuSe* to draw a clinical picture of the patient is its ability to bring together and display information about the complex dynamic interactions between the physical, social, experiential, conceptual, and narrative facets of the self.

A focus on the physical facet of *MuSe* might also yield information about how long the individual has been exposed to a particular substance, with important implications for interventions. For example, while alcohol dependency can take months or years after the initial sampling, opioids can cause physical dependence after a very short period of use (four to eight weeks) (Fidler et al. 2006, 30). In fact, the rapid development of dependency constitutes one of the biggest challenges to recovery from OUD, as an abrupt stop, even after a short period of use, leads to severe withdrawal effects, including generalized pain, chills, cramps, restlessness, anxiety, nausea, vomiting, insomnia, and very intense cravings. The withdrawal effects may feel insurmountable, and the individual may eventually give up and start using again. For this reason, abstinence-based programs that are dominant in the United States and Canada have poor outcomes. Many overdose deaths in the context of OUD occur after periods of withdrawal. Similarly, individuals with problematic alcohol use patterns experience heightened levels of anxiety, restlessness, and irritability when their consumption is delayed. When they attempt to quit drinking, their hands may shake, and they may become anxious, restless, and irritable. They may experience sleep disturbances and anxiety, waking up in the middle of the night with nausea or with a desire to consume alcohol. In fact, the craving may be "the only tune or story in the addict's head, and nothing else drives it out" (Graham 2013, 178). At times, individuals may experience life-threatening symptoms such as delirium and hallucinations. Here, for example, the clinician may explain the individual's patterns of withdrawal and craving to them via the brain disease framework, while cautioning them that the research is ongoing, and substance use patterns have important relationships with non-physical aspects of life. Be that as it may, the metabolization of the drug of choice by the body and its influence on the brain can be important in making sense of the physical mechanisms underlying SUDs. Ultimately, using *MuSe*, a clinician might ask questions that will extract information about the physical facet of the individual's experience and set this within the context of information drawn from the trilateral strategy, thus suggesting what strategy might help this particular person.

The *social facet* of *MuSe* provides an entry into the involvement of sociality in an individual's substance use patterns and can suggest possible intervention strategies when used in conjunction with the trilateral strategy. With the help of insights gained by using the trilateral strategy, the clinician already knows social relationships of care and concern are instrumental in the formation, enrichment, or impoverishment of the self, and substance use often represents a response to things not going very well in the individual's social life. Individuals in unhappy relationships often report seeking refuge in alcohol consumption or opioid use. Drugs, thus serve a purpose. In addition, ample scientific research shows complex family histories involving trauma or physical or sexual abuse as a child are strongly linked to SUD (Marcenko et al. 2000; Langeland et al. 2002). Similarly, substance use habits develop in a particular kind of social environment. Consider, for example, "the male life of public and gregarious heavy drinking" outlined by Owen Flanagan, where the drug use becomes the primary context through which individuals socialize in their professional lives (Flanagan 2013b, 870). A causal drink after a business meeting might turn into the sole reason to go to the meeting.

In turn, existing social or interpersonal problems may be exacerbated by the effects of the opioid. Often the individual fails to meet the responsibilities of care and concern for others—the building blocks of healthy interpersonal and work relationships. This leads to further isolation from the community, loss of job and social status, etc., aggravating the abuse patterns. Engaging with the patient in a way that acquires information about the social facet of *MuSe* is important, as it yields information about the role of social relationships in the development of the individual's use of substances. Armed with this knowledge and using the trilateral strategy, the clinician can direct the individual towards more empowering social relationships. A clinician might ask whether the individual consumes the substance alone, if the habit started in response to a social situation, how loved ones respond, and so on. Then, the clinician can use this information about the social facet in a way that connects it to the other facets of *MuSe*, streamlining the complexity of the individual's experience to facilitate interventions.

In response to the clinician's exploration of the *experiential facet* of *MuSe*, the individual might describe the lived experience of the desire for the drug, cravings for the drug, the distress of not using it when consumption is delayed, and regrets about consuming it despite resolutions to the contrary. As discussed previously, the experiential aspect of *MuSe* (such as feelings of pain) is not immediately available to anyone other than the experiencing subject, but the use of *MuSe* by the clinician can reveal crucial information about these experiences. It is valuable to probe the individual in a way that will help them express what it is like to encounter the pull of substances. For example, Caroline Knapp describes drinking alone (individuals with SUDs often do this to hide their drinking from others) as entering into a room of one's own and closing the blinds, turning inwards. She writes that the alcohol becomes the only company she enjoys; her mood changes, and "the awfulness settles" with the first drink. The first drink leads to other drinks and drunkenness. The next day she hates herself again. The cycle repeats (Knapp 1996). Clinicians who are equipped with information gathered through the linguistic representation of these experiences (from testimonies) can use the information to develop interventions that will enhance agency and autonomy. More specifically, when *MuSe* is used in conjunction with the trilateral strategy, the clinician can probe the individual about their experiences, habits, and self-related feelings, trying to help them articulate their experiences in a way that will enable them to understand their patterns of thoughts and behavior and develop skills that may be helpful next time they are in a similar state. In addition, accumulating information about the experiential facet might suggest novel targets to scientifically investigate and track what kinds of interventions may or may not help individuals. As we better understand the experiential facet of substance use patterns and distresses, we might be able to understand what successful interventions look like.

The *narrative facet* of *MuSe* offers a helpful medium to engage with an individual with SUD. As outlined in the previous chapters, the processes involved in the narrative facet track the individual's perception of their lives as a whole, including how they make sense of their past and its relationship to their present and future, how they started using, how problematic substance use patterns developed, and how these experiences interact with other facets of their lives. In fact, much of the work that goes into recovery involves the individual's reconciliation of different and sometimes conflicting life narratives into a more or less coherent one. For example, an individual's social identity can be a central part of how they developed SUD and why they continue to consume the drug despite its severe negative consequences (Pickard 2021). As Pickard argues, it is hard to explain many cases of substance use related behavior without recognizing the *value* of drugs to individuals. Thus, the clinician's probing of and engagement with the patient's self-narrative might guide the patient to merge multiple and sometimes conflicting narratives into one that is more aligned with the kind of narrative the patient wants to live and tell.

Such kinds of narrative conflict and adjudication can be found in David Foster Wallace's account of his experience in a halfway house following his hospitalization for SUD when he was 27 (Max 2013). The realities of the halfway house, including what he needed to do to follow the program to stop using substances and the social environment, were quite different from his own realities. Until his hospitalization and transition to the halfway house, Wallace's life narrative centered on his identity as a famous author, his struggles and successes in writing, his enrollment in Harvard to do a PhD in philosophy, etc. All these self-narratives featured the identity of an intellectual who has the financial and educational privilege to live as an author. Suddenly, in the halfway house, he was expected to find "low-level work" as a security guard and share a barracks-like room with four men who had "a tattoo or a criminal record or both!" (Max 2013) Wallace was self-reportedly humiliated and confused, as his own image and narrative of his life did not synch with the narrative he was now placed in, i.e., that of an individual recovering from SUD in a halfway house he shared with people otherwise very different from him. D.T. Max writes in his biography of Wallace that he:

> "knew it was imperative to abandon the sense of himself as the smartest person in the room, a person too smart to be like one of the people in the room, because he was one of the people in the room."
>
> (Max 2013)

Part of Wallace's story of his recovery and return to writing owes to his adjudication of these conflicts within his self-narratives. In the midst of "his misery," as Max points out, Wallace was alive to the new information he was acquiring from his social environment, and his observations of his fellow residents in the halfway house, along with his self-reflections, led him to start writing again, and this, at least briefly, was helpful for his recovery.

The *conceptual facet* of *MuSe* is also revelatory of the individual's experience with substance use, as it displays how the individual thinks about themselves. An individual's self-concepts are formed in the process of the dynamic interaction between the self and the physical, social, and cultural environments. They emerge from the individual's perceptions of their physical body, social relationships, and narratives about life experiences. They also draw on the features of the physical, social, and cultural environment. For example, an individual's self-concept as a "dedicated father" is the product of the social facet of his selfhood and the norms of being a dedicated parent in a specific culture. Another important feature of self-concepts is that they can shape the self as a whole because they are action-guiding (Tekin 2014a, 2015). They inform how individuals behave and relate to their relationships and environment, sometimes even motivating them to change. For example, my idea of myself as a swimmer might propel me to train with a group of triathletes, and this, in turn, might enhance my self-concept as a good swimmer. Importantly, positive and resourceful self-concepts expand the individual's possibilities for action (Jopling 2000; Tekin 2011, 2015).

As I have discussed in Chapter 4, self-concepts are informed by mental distresses and disorders to which the individual is subjected and by the ways these are framed in medical and social contexts. This influence is mediated, first, by the changes that occur in the physical and social facets of the self, owing to distress or disorders, second, by the scientifically based or folk-psychological knowledge available to the individual about their condition, and third, by their self-narratives in which they make sense of their condition (Tekin 2011, 2014a, 2014b, 2014c, 2015). Therefore, approaching an individual with problematic substance use patterns through the conceptual dimension of *MuSe*, in conjunction with the trilateral strategy, provides resources for interventions. Consider the following scenario. A person's heavy consumption of substances might mean they cannot keep their promises, which might, in turn, negatively affect their relationships, exacerbating the problematic substance use pattern. A father may promise to watch his daughter play soccer yet not make it to the practice because he is heavily intoxicated. Failing to follow through on promises and disappointing his loved ones, when repeated over time, may alter his self-concept as a reliable person or a dedicated father. He may develop feelings of frustration or even hatred of himself. He may decide to stop making promises or even taking on responsibilities that require keeping promises. However, these self-concepts, when engaged in the clinical context, might be very helpful for the clinician. The clinician may realize what is actually important for him, i.e., being a good father, and encourage and motivate him to change in order to have more positive self-concepts.

In fact, self-regarding attitudes, such as bewilderment, disappointment, and shame, are among the core features of the experience of problematic substance use (Flanagan 2013a, 6). Consider relapse, for example. People struggling with substance use often refrain from the addictive behavior during certain periods but do not always achieve lasting success. They "fall back" into the detrimental behavior after a temporary stoppage. After the relapse, the individual might self-interpret themselves as a failure, and relapse becomes a source of shame, regret, self-blame, and embarrassment, as well as diminished self-confidence and self-esteem. These experiences influence the individual's self-concept: for example, the individual may think they lack self-discipline. Because self-concepts are not just descriptive but also prescriptive, they inform how individuals behave and can motivate them to change. In the context of SUD, self-concepts form or influence future actions. Hopelessness in the face of repeated relapses and self-concepts such as being weak-willed may diminish a person's ability to end the addictive behavior. Alternatively, they may express conflict and heightened distress because of a strong resolution to quit drinking, especially if they are unable to do so. From this conflict, they can redefine themselves and their behavioral goals consistent with that self-concept. They may take a step towards change, altering their self-concept and stabilizing the new behavior pattern. In addition, perceiving themselves as someone who needs help, they may reach out to communities of other individuals with SUD. The success of AA programs partly owes to this.

In clinical contexts, the information on the individual's social self-concepts can be used as a hook to motivate them to work on their consumption in a sustainable manner over the long term. Using the trilateral strategy, clinicians can work with the individual to develop realistic and resourceful self-concepts so they can change their relationship with the substance and strengthen their agency and autonomy. In addition, understanding the relationship between drug consumption and self-concepts may help the individual acquire psychological and social skills, further enhancing autonomy and agency.

7.4 *MuSe* and SUD among veterans

In a recent study, my colleagues and I examined the explanatory resourcefulness of *MuSe* in predicting SUD diagnosis status among veterans by leveraging a nationwide survey of post-9/11 veterans receiving regular Department of Veterans Affairs (VA) care (Tekin et al. 2022). We used existing survey and medical record data curated from the Trajectories of Resilience and Comorbidity Clusters in Operations Enduring Freedom and Iraqi Freedom Veterans (TRACC OEF-OIF) and performed a secondary analysis of the data by examining each of the five domains/facets of *MuSe* (see Table 7.1).[1] SUD diagnoses were identified using the diagnostic codes

Table 7.1 Description of data elements from the nationwide post-9/11 veteran survey relative to *MuSe* domains.

Multitudinous Self Model domain	Measure used	Description
Physical	Diagnosis codes for mental and physical health conditions	Indicates presence of a post-traumatic stress disorder, depression, anxiety, insomnia, pain, or hypertension/high blood pressure diagnosis in the medical record.
Social	Military-to-Civilian Questionnaire (M2CQ)	Measures difficulty with post-deployment community reintegration following separation from military service.
Experiential	Patient Health Questionnaire 15-item version (PHQ-15)	Measures severity of common somatic symptoms reported in clinical care.
Narrative	Question regarding emotional health over time	A single question asks the respondent to compare emotional health now to emotional health one year ago.
Conceptual	Self-Efficacy for Life Tasks (SELT)	Measures perceived confidence in the ability to complete developmentally appropriate life tasks (e.g., hold down a job, take care of family).

used during clinical care. To conservatively identify SUD diagnoses, we only included cases with one inpatient diagnosis or two outpatient diagnoses at least seven days apart.

To measure the *physical facet,* we looked at the recorded diagnostic codes for the veterans, including both mental and physical health conditions. These indicated whether the individual had a diagnosis of a post-traumatic stress disorder, depression, anxiety, insomnia, pain, or hypertension/high blood pressure diagnosis in their medical record. To measure the *social facet,* we used a Military-to-Civilian Questionnaire (M2CQ) which identified difficulties with post-deployment community reintegration following separation from military service. To explore the *experiential facet,* we used the Patient Health Questionnaire (PHQ-15) measuring the severity of common somatic symptoms reported in clinical care. For the *narrative facet,* we looked at veterans' answers to a question on emotional health over time. More specifically, veterans were asked to compare their emotional health now to their health one year ago. Finally, to measure the *conceptual facet,* we looked at the results of the Self-Efficacy for Life Tasks (SELT) survey. The SELT provided insights into veterans' perceived confidence in their ability to complete developmentally appropriate life tasks (e.g., hold down a job, take care of family).

Each domain of *MuSe* significantly predicted SUD diagnoses when entered into separate univariate models (all ps < 0.01). In other words, self-related phenomena individuated by each facet of *MuSe* were found to play a causal role in an individual's SUD. For the physical facet, each mental and physical diagnosis was associated with greater odds of SUD diagnoses. Mental health diagnoses (i.e., post-traumatic stress disorder, depression, and anxiety) had the strongest statistical association with SUD diagnoses. This has important implications for the multimorbidity of mental disorders, as it suggests self-related phenomena are fundamentally at play in different mental disorders. In the social facet, difficulty with community reintegration measured using the military-to-civilian question also predicted the likelihood of SUD diagnoses; the worse the social integration post-deployment, the higher the likelihood of veterans being diagnosed with SUD. In the experiential facet, veterans who reported more somatic symptoms on the PHQ-15 were significantly more likely to have SUD diagnoses while in VA care, and in the narrative facet, veterans who indicated their emotional health had declined in the preceding year were more likely to have SUD diagnoses. Finally, in the conceptual facet, veterans' confidence in their self-efficacy to complete developmentally appropriate life tasks as indicated by the SELT was associated with diminished frequency of SUD diagnoses. These findings indicate that each of the facets of *MuSe* is associated with the development and maintenance of SUD. However, when all these factors were simultaneously entered into a logistic regression model predicting SUD diagnoses, only the social, experiential, and conceptual domains remained significant predictors (Tekin et al. 2022).

As our work suggests, facets of *MuSe* can help track substance use problems; as such, it is an empirically responsive model that can be used in scientific research in psychiatry. Importantly, our work highlights the unique value of social support even after accounting for mental health diagnoses; this finding offers possible resources for clinicians who are treating individuals and for the individuals themselves who are trying to overcome SUD.

This preliminary study is by no means conclusive about the explanatory power of *MuSe*, nor does it determine precisely which interventions lead to flourishing. However, it does show the model is aligned with testimonial and clinical expertise on SUDs and their care and thus has implications for scientific research. Our analysis of the data on SUD among veterans resulted in two important conclusions with a bearing on the development of interventions that will aid flourishing. First, SUDs among veterans are associated with the existence of other mental health problems, such as anxiety, depression, and post-traumatic stress disorder. Second, better community reintegration after military service is associated with reduced SUD diagnoses, suggesting social connections may be critical factors in positive outcomes. While it is not possible to extricate from our data whether reduced social support is vulnerable to or a negative consequence of SUD diagnoses, our findings underscore the need to account for social support as a matter of standard clinical care. Enhanced education on or access to social programs that can bolster emotional, social, and tangible support resources could benefit all veterans, but may particularly aid those struggling with substance use. In this sense, models that make the social dimensions of these conditions central, such as *MuSe*, are likely to guide the systematic development of strategies to generate social support in the treatment of SUD, unlike the brain disease model, which does not focus on social determinants of mental health.

Our study has broader significance for philosophy of science and cognitive science in so far as it invites philosophers of psychiatry to engage in empirical research on subjects previously examined from the armchair. This empirical move should be situated in the recent methodological debates on the value of traditional conceptual analysis in philosophy (Machery 2017; Strevens 2019). Broadly defined, traditional conceptual analysis is the method of answering a philosophical question such as "What is disease?" by analyzing relevant concepts, such as "being treated by medical professionals" or "experiencing distress." The relevant concept, i.e., "being treated by medical professionals," is then analyzed using thought experiments or counterexamples. The result of this process is the determination of the necessary and sufficient conditions for a phenomenon to be called "disease." For example, we may realize that defining "disease" as "a condition treated by medical professionals" is wrong, as conditions such as pregnancy are treated by medical professionals but fail to fall under the category of "disease." In this sense, a thought experiment or a counterexample could provide suggestive evidence showing the insufficiency of some of the properties.

Traditional conceptual analysis has been called into question for a variety of reasons by feminist philosophers, empirically informed philosophers, and experimental philosophers. Feminist scholars have criticized traditional concepts such as knowledge as justified true belief, arguing instead for embodied and situated knowledge (e.g., Code 1991). Similarly, as discussed in Chapter 4, empirically informed philosophers of mind have proposed the Real People Challenge (Tekin 2021), expressing concerns about the over-reliance on thought experiments or counterexamples in conceptual analysis at the expense of engaging with real-world phenomena.

Experimental philosophers have joined these criticisms of traditional conceptual analyses by arguing concepts do not have a definitional structure, and there is variation in the intuitions used to test proposed analyses and counterexamples. They call for a naturalized conceptual analysis that engages with and is responsive to empirical research and real-world frameworks (Machery 2017). Naturalized conceptual analysis requires empirical methods to be pursued successfully for philosophers to arrive at knowledge that is "within their epistemic reach" (Machery 2017). These methods include 1) generating actual empirical knowledge in the domains where these concepts do epistemic work; and 2) conducting studies in experimental philosophy.

The study we conducted on the explanatory power of *MuSe* falls under 1), in the sense that we generated empirical knowledge on how well the model could explain the connection between veterans' complex selfhood and their substance use (Tekin et al. 2022). Naturalized conceptual analysis is epistemically beneficial because it helps philosophers identify concepts that are invalid, obscure, or ambiguous. In Machery's view, what follows conceptual analysis is conceptual engineering, defined as the modification of an existing concept in light of naturalized conceptual analysis. The goal of conceptual engineering is to remedy the epistemic flaws in concepts, such as obscurity, imprecision, etc.

I believe the philosophy of psychiatry would benefit from naturalized conceptual analysis (Tekin 2023). Such a discussion is beyond the scope of this book, but my hope is that studies like ours might be instrumental in clarifying what the self is—in a metaphysical sense—and in determining whether *MuSe* provides a scaffolding for how to think about interventions that lead to flourishing.

7.5 *MuSe*, OUD, and flourishing

MuSe provides valuable resources for both the individuals diagnosed with SUD and the clinicians treating them. Clinicians might offer better treatments by engaging with the five facets of *MuSe* and using the trilateral strategy. At the same time, active engagement with the five facets of *MuSe* might help the individual better understand their substance use patterns, empower them to take an active part in their recovery through a multi-pronged engagement with the self and ultimately flourish.

One advantage of understanding SUD in relation to *MuSe* is the model's focus on flourishing rather than full recovery—which is often taken to be complete abstinence from substances. Under *MuSe*, it is plausible to consider that an individual might enhance their agency and autonomy, even if they do not fully abstain. I now take a closer look at a non-standard but fairly successful treatment method for OUD, substitution therapy (in lieu of abstinence-based approaches), and argue its success can be attributed to its engagement with the fundamental features of *MuSe* and its use of a trilateral strategy.

Opioids are a class of drugs that derive from or mimic substances found in opium poppy plants. They produce a variety of effects in the brain, including pain reduction or relief, by activating nerve cells in a way that blocks pain signals. Examples of opioids include morphine, heroin, codeine, oxycodone, hydrocodone, and fentanyl. Some opioids are prescription pain medicine, and others circulate as illegal drugs. The United States and Canada are seeing crises of OUD and overdose deaths. According to a report from the US Center for Disease Control's National Center for Health Statistics, an estimated 107,543 people died of drug overdoses in 2023; 81,023 of these deaths involved opioids (National Center for Health Statistics 2024). Effective interventions are sorely needed.

An unconventional and fairly controversial (at least in North America) OUD treatment is substitution therapy. Substitution therapy, also called "agonist pharmacotherapy," "agonist replacement therapy," and "agonist-assisted therapy," is defined as:

> ... the administration under medical supervision of a prescribed psychoactive substance, pharmacologically related to the one producing dependence, to people with substance dependence, for achieving defined treatment aims. Substitution therapy is widely used in the management of nicotine ("nicotine replacement therapy") and opioid dependence.
> (World Health Organization, 2004)

Current treatments for OUD include a spectrum of abstinence-based approaches, the core principle of which is fully stopping the consumption of the drug with which the individual has problems, and substitution therapy approaches, in which the individual receives a very low dose of the drug under supervision on a regular schedule. A typical example of an abstinence-based approach is the strict no-alcohol principle of AA groups. An example of substitution therapy is methadone maintenance therapy, in which the patient receives injectable opioids under supervised conditions. The main goals of substitution therapy are to prevent overdose deaths, manage the (challenging) withdrawal process, and enable the individual to have better life quality. Substitution therapy interventions involve giving the patient tapered methadone or buprenorphine/naloxone while simultaneously providing psychosocial interventions. Therapy comes in various forms, depending on the kind of opioid prescribed, and it requires supervised conditions.

One form of substitution therapy is heroin-assisted treatment (HAT), in which patients with a long-term, treatment-refractory OUD are prescribed injectable diacetylmorphine—the active ingredient of heroin. A tremendous body of scientific evidence shows the effectiveness of HAT (Ferri et al. 2010; Oviedo-Joekes et al. 2016; Strang et al. 2015). HAT is widely used in European countries, including Denmark, Germany, Luxembourg, the Netherlands, and the United Kingdom, but this form of treatment or even conducting research on it is illegal in Canada and the United States because diacetylmorphine and heroin are illegal. Interestingly, the DSM-5 describes maintenance therapy as a form of intervention to address OUD, but it does not recognize diacetylmorphine or heroin as opioids that could be used in maintenance therapy. According to the DSM-5, maintenance therapy involves "taking a prescribed agonist medication such as methadone or buprenorphine" (American Psychiatric Association 2022). Heroin-assisted treatment is not discussed as a treatment option in the class of maintenance therapy (for more on this, see Steel and Tekin 2021).

Data on patients who have received HAT show the intervention improves their quality of life and contributes to their flourishing, in so far as it helps them develop capacities that enhance their agency and autonomy. The primary reason for the success of substitution therapy, including HAT, I argue, is its direct engagement with the complexity of the individual's selfhood and its use of the trilateral strategy in the sense that it gives uptake to patients' expertise and demonstrates rigorous engagement with up-to-date scientific and clinical data.

Consider the results of two studies. The North American Opiate Medication Initiative (NAOMI) running from 2005 to 2008 was the first clinical trial of prescribed heroin in North America. NAOMI was an open, randomized, controlled trial comparing injected diacetylmorphine with oral methadone alone in the treatment of OUD (Oviedo-Joekes et al. 2008). Participants were injection opioid users who had not benefited from other therapies. The results showed patients treated with injectable diacetylmorphine were more likely to stay in treatment and more likely to reduce their use of illegal drugs and other illegal activities than patients treated with oral methadone.

During the NAOMI study, researchers provided injectable hydromorphone, a licensed pain medication, to a small group of participants. An unexpected finding was that many participants could not tell the difference between the effects of diacetylmorphine, the active ingredient of heroin, and hydromorphone. The small number of participants receiving hydromorphone was insufficient for researchers to draw any definite and scientifically valid conclusions on its efficacy as a treatment option.

The second study, the Study to Assess Long-term Opioid Maintenance Effectiveness (SALOME), tested alternative treatments for people with chronic heroin addiction who were currently not benefiting sufficiently from available treatments such as oral methadone (Oviedo-Joekes et al. 2016). SALOME was a three-year, double-blind, non-inferiority trial comparing the effectiveness of diacetylmorphine and hydromorphone. This trial study was considered important, because if hydromorphone was found to be as effective as diacetylmorphine, the benefits of this type of treatment might be achievable without the legal barriers and stigma associated with heroin. SALOME participants were long-term street opioid users and represented the minority of individuals with severe OUD who had not benefited from first-line addiction treatments such as oral methadone. On average, they had been injecting street heroin for about 15 years. They had attempted methadone maintenance therapy at least twice in the past five years but had not succeeded. Sixty percent were homeless.

SALOME involved two stages. Each trial participant remained in each stage for six months. In stage one, half of the 202 participants were randomized to receive injectable diacetylmorphine, while the other half received injectable hydromorphone. This was a double-blind study—neither the participants nor the researchers and clinical team (other than the pharmacy) knew which treatment was being administered. In stage two, half of the participants were randomized to continue injection treatment exactly as in stage one, while the other half switched to the oral equivalent of the same medication (diacetylmorphine or hydromorphone). The oral version was also provided on a double-blind basis. SALOME concluded in 2015, and the results were published in April 2016 (Oviedo-Joekes et al. 2016).

Once in the study, participants visited the clinic up to three times per day; after a pre-treatment assessment (for safety reasons), they received their medication. After injecting or ingesting their medication, they were observed until staff determined it was safe for them to leave. Physicians specializing in OUD monitored the prescriptions for both groups. In addition, throughout the treatment period, an interdisciplinary team of physicians, nurses, social workers, and counselors was available to help participants achieve stability in their lives, seek employment, and find suitable housing. Some primary care services, as well as HIV, hepatitis C, and psychiatric care, were provided. At any time, participants could choose to switch to methadone treatment, to drug-free (abstinence) programs, to detox programs, or to any other option available. A research team conducted individual assessments to determine if the treatments were effective. This team worked closely with but independently from the clinical team and had no power over clinical decisions.

Findings showed hydromorphone was as effective as diacetylmorphine in treating severe OUD. This means that in jurisdictions where diacetylmorphine is not available for legal reasons, hydromorphone could be offered as a licensed alternative. Participants on both medications reported far fewer days of street heroin and other opioid use at six months (three to five days per month), compared to almost daily illicit opioid use prior to being enrolled in the study. They also reported a significant reduction in days of illegal activities (from an average of 14.1 days per month to less than four).

The versions of substitution therapy used in NAOMI and SALOME engaged with all facets of *MuSe*. This integrated approach to the complexity of OUD was more successful than single-metric interventions.

First, engagement with the physical facet of *MuSe* was key to success. As illustrated in the NAOMI and SALOME trials, as well as prior European studies, the supervised long-term substitution of methadone and buprenorphine can reduce or in some cases eliminate OUD (West and Brown 2013, 32). From this perspective, the primary tasks of treatment are to: 1) identify the specific needs the substance is being used to meet (e.g., to be able to fall asleep); 2) develop skills that provide alternative ways of meeting those needs; and 3) use these drugs to supplement the person's transition from heroin addiction to more resourceful and less harmful ways of meeting their needs.

The biggest source of success for the SALOME study was its ability to control the withdrawal effects of opioid dependence among individuals who had not responded to other forms of maintenance therapy. The right formula of the medication kept people stable and did not push them to overdose or use street drugs. One SALOME participant said the study offered "people like us, lifelong addicts, a chance to perhaps begin to 'MANAGE' our addiction with a degree of success" (Supporters of Salome 2017). He said he was "off all pills," "no longer on the streets," and had his "first home" after "eight and a half years in jail." Thanks to the regimented reception, he knew what drug he was taking and was "not risking [his] life by doing fentanyl" (Supporters of Salome 2017).

Another participant wrote:

> This program has worked for me by saving my life. When I started I was overweight and on 17 different pills for a variety of different stuff from arthritis to a heart condition. Plus supporting two habits from heroin to crack; now I am off all pills. I am no longer on the streets. I have got my first home. I'm single for the first time in my addict life. My life in a nutshell.
>
> (Supporters of Salome 2017)

What is particularly remarkable in the self-report above is the writer's conviction that they were not able to exercise any kind of agency, owing to their dependency, but a regimented and routine consumption of drugs in a supervised environment gave them a certain kind of control over their actions and structure in their lives.

Other self-reports from SALOME participants reflected similar transformations in agency and autonomy. For example, one participant described the physical development of the opioid dependency and explained how it was later subdued:

> I have been a member since almost day one. I believe I was the fourth client enrolled. I'm slightly different than others have in that I am an addict however I also live my life in pain. I was born with spinal bifida, so this program allows me to walk and work and be somewhat functional. I was able to go back to college for two years and study community mental health and addictions worker. I'm now employed as peer supervisor in the chill at insight injection facility. I stay active in the community fundraising and obtaining grants to host numerous projects around the downtown Eastside. in contrast this is a very different lifestyle I am living compared to pre-crosstown clinic where I was forced onto methadone forced out of work ultimately forced onto assistance and forced to live downtown Eastside. ... In short, I don't know how anyone could not recognize this program as a recovery base program ... sadly many of the abstinence programs have long missed ... on this one. Having spent 10 years in an auto recovery for cocaine addiction, coupled with owning and operating my own recovery houses, I take a different approach. I believe in teaching to be functional first, [then] abstinence if necessary.
>
> (Supporters of Salome 2017)

Finally, participants observed the deadly consequences of OUDs and recognized a regimented and supervised intake during the SALOME trial saved their lives. As one commented, the people in this program "have tried other treatment options, to no avail, continued failure, ongoing cycle, jails, institutions and finally death" (Supporters of Salome 2017). Another participant pointed to overdose deaths, suggesting the urgent need to develop programs like SALOME: "The drugs on the street are so much stronger and insanely potent that people on the street are overdosing and dropping like flies" (Supporters of Salome 2017).

Second, the SALOME study engaged with the social facet of *MuSe* and addressed OUD thorough an emphasis on social relationships. It enhanced individuals' social relationships by helping them connect with others who shared the same experience. A participant in the SALOME trials said the program "has given [my] dignity back ... without having to hustle for the next fix on the street" (Supporters of Salome 2017). The participant said they "made friends in the clinic, those who face the same barriers ... in maintaining a healthy lifestyle and we support each other through hard times and good" (Supporters of Salome 2017). Having a good support network during recovery strengthened participants' ability to stick with the treatment plan. Another participant said that since joining the program, they had not been "in trouble with the law," adding, "No more in and out of jail. That cycle door has stopped" (Supporters of Salome 2017). Thanks to the SALOME trial, they had their "life back."

The social facet of *MuSe* highlights the need for socially based interventions. For example, SALOME engaged with participants to understand how they perceived their trajectory in treatment. Mimicking the fundamental commitment of the trilateral strategy to testimonials, researchers published a series of letters written by the participants on their progress. One participant recorded the transition from living with opioid dependency to living a more regulated life beyond drug use:

Being an addict for the past 30 years off and on. Trying different treatments for no avail, the methadone and so forth. The end is always the same, jails, institutions, and death. Having been involved in Crosstown Clinic for the past three years it has done what no other place could. Seeing what fentanyl has done I am glad I was a client at Cross Town Clinic. ... [T]his new drug has been brought around. The chances would be very good that I would first be a rather statistic. ... To have more clinics like Crosstown, could you imagine how many of our friends would still be alive. Hoping to see more of our Health Care budget put to good use on this War on the drug fentanyl. How many more have to die?

(Supporters of Salome 2017)

Autobiographical insights like these suggest tools for treating other patients with similar experiences.

Third, SALOME tapped into the experiential and narrative facets of *MuSe*, in that it used participants' ability to evaluate the trajectory of their experience with opioid use. They were encouraged to reflectively engage with their experience of repetitive use, followed by feelings of regret, followed by a resolve to quit but an inability to do so, owing to withdrawal effects. Relief from the withdrawal effects gave them the space to think about the circumstances in which they were more prone to using (social settings). Reflective engagement is also used in therapies that teach patients "stimulus control strategies." In these therapies, patients learn to avoid situations associated with drug use and to spend more time in activities incompatible with drug use. They practice "urge control" by recognizing and changing the thoughts, feelings, and plans that lead to drug use. Patients' past attempts and failures are used as a benchmark to customize the therapy (Azrin et al. 1994a, 1994b). A qualitative study on the SALOME participants' experiences with the treatment highlighted significant improvement in health. Many of the participants reported they improved their nutrition and reduced their stress and risky behavior, such as sex work (Jozaghi 2014). A participant, Joe, said he used to be in pain and was constantly in and out of hospital, but the program helped him manage his pain and gave him more energy (Jozaghi 2014).

Fourth, SALOME focused on participants' self-concepts, the conceptual facet of *MuSe*. As I have discussed in previous chapters, because of their plastic nature, self-concepts offer great opportunities for successful clinical interventions. SALOME enabled participants to develop more positive and resourceful self-concepts, boosting their self-esteem. Their self-reports revealed the gradual strengthening of self-governance and self-concepts. One participant said that before the trial, their life was "unstable," and they "could not plan anything," as their "future was a big void." They were not sure if their future was going to be sickness, jail, or death in a back alley. The SALOME study "saved" them, because with the supervised use of low-dose drugs, the sickness associated with withdrawals was gone. The participant was able to focus on other things like looking for a job. Their health improved, and they could "better take care of" themselves. They were able to nurture other "plusses" in their life, and they started seeing themselves in a more positive light, as able to take care of themselves (Supporters of Salome 2017). Another participant noted that prior to SALOME, they were just a "thief and a criminal," but now, post-SALOME, they are "clean" and have gone to college. They can "work and buy nice things," and they "feel free" (Supporters of Salome 2017).

Notably, the substitution therapy illustrated in the SALOME study inches closer to the expansive notions of expertise and objectivity promoted by *MuSe* and the trilateral strategy in that the study included patients not only as "objects" of psychiatric research but also as subjects. In addition to assessing the effectiveness of the substitution therapy through metrics such as urine tests or observations of behavior, researchers asked participants about their perceptions of their treatment and recovery. To that end, they collected letters from participants about their experience in the study and the effects they observed. In addition, SALOME administered a survey on the perceived effectiveness of the program. A huge majority, 91.6 percent, said the treatment they were receiving was effective; only 5.2 percent said it was not, and 3.1 percent were unsure. The most commonly cited reasons for reported effectiveness were improved health, improved quality of life, and reduced or halted street drug use, with a similar proportion of men and women referencing these themes. This was a notable outcome because results from the NAOMI trial showed many trial participants were drawn to the treatment because of the possibility of receiving pharmaceutical-grade heroin. However, there was *not* a strong emphasis on the medication itself when SALOME participants explained why the treatment was effective for them. Instead, they spoke of improvements in various aspects of life, including interpersonal relationships, health, and quality of life—areas they said they were able to focus on once their physical dependence was addressed.

These initial efforts to actively involve participants in research have generated some post-trial and participant-generated research and activism. Because it was only during the SALOME trial that the patients were able to receive hydromorphone and diacetylmorphine injections, they came together as a group post-trial to increase awareness of the effectiveness of these interventions and to lobby the Canadian government to legalize them. They formed the SALOME/NAOMI Association of Patients (SNAP), a peer-run group of former research participants, and developed research principles using the critical methodological frameworks on community-based research for social justice (Boyd et al. 2017). Note that the formation of this group and their research and activism efforts are great examples of the inclusion of patients as experts in research frameworks. In an article coauthored by researchers and experience-based experts, they highlight areas of concern, including "life prior to SALOME," "clinic setting and routine," "stability," "6-month transition," "support," "exiting the trial and ethics," and "collective action" (Boyd et al. 2017). Based on this work, the group launched a constitutional challenge in the Supreme Court of British Colombia to continue receiving opioid-assisted treatments after the SALOME trial ended. They also advocated for the creation of alternative harm reduction programs throughout Canada. As this case suggests, it is essential to recognize patients as knowers, as experts who must play a fundamental role in generating knowledge on mental disorders and their treatment.

7.6 Conclusion

This chapter explained how *MuSe*, in conjunction with the trilateral strategy integrating testimonial, scientific, and clinical knowledge, can create resources for individuals with SUD to flourish. Section 2 examined how the brain disease model of SUD engages with individuals with substance use problems. Section 3 juxtaposed the *MuSe*-based framework to the brain disease model of SUD, highlighting how *MuSe* offers comparatively more clinical and reflective resources. Section 4 gave a brief overview of a study evaluating the explanatory power of *MuSe* in understanding SUD among veterans. Section 5 discussed substitution therapy, a controversial method to address OUD, arguing this form of treatment is more successful than abstinence-based therapies because it demonstrates a deep engagement with the fundamental aspects of *MuSe* and adopts a trilateral strategy combining scientific, clinical, and experiential knowledge.

Note

1 At the time of the study, the names of the facets of the Multitudinous Self Model were as follows: ecological, intersubjective, private, temporally extended, and conceptual. These have since been replaced by physical, social, experiential, narrative, and conceptual. The name changes do not affect the analysis or the outcomes of the study.

References

American Psychiatric Association. 2022. *Diagnostic and Statistical Manual of Mental Disorders: DSM-5-TR*. American Psychiatric Association Publishing.
Azrin, N.H., B. Donohue, V.A. Besalel, E.S. Kogan, and R. Acierno. 1994a. Youth Drug Abuse Treatment: A Controlled Outcome Study. *Journal of Child and Adolescent Substance Use* 3(3), 1–16.
Azrin, N.H., P.T. McMahon, B. Donahue, V. Besalel, K.J. Lapinski, E. Kogan, et al. 1994b. Behavioral Therapy for Drug Abuse: A Controlled Treatment Outcome Study. *Behavioral Research and Therapy* 32(8), 857–866.
Boyd, Susan, Dave Murray, SNAP, and Donald MacPherson. 2017. "Telling Our Stories: Heroin-Assisted Treatment and SNAP Activism in the Downtown Eastside of Vancouver." *Harm Reduction Journal* 14(27). doi:10.1186/s12954-017-0152-3.
Code, Lorraine. 1991. *What Can She Know? Feminist Theory and the Construction of Knowledge*. Ithaca, NY: Cornell University Press.
Ferri, Marica, Marina Davoli, and Carlo A. Perucci. 2010. Heroin Maintenance for Chronic Heroin-Dependent Individuals. *Cochrane Database of Systematic Reviews* 8. doi:10.1002/14651858.CD003410.pub3.
Fidler, Tara L., Tara W. Clews, and Christopher L. Cunningham. 2006. Reestablishing an Intragastric Ethanol Self-Infusion Model in Rats. *Alcoholism: Clinical and Experimental Research* 30(3), 414–428. doi:10.1111/j.1530-0277.2006.00046.x.
Flanagan, Owen. 2013a. Identity and Addiction: What Alcoholic Memoirs Teach. In *The Oxford Handbook of Philosophy and Psychiatry*, edited by K.W.M. Fulford,

M. Davies, R. Gipps, G. Graham, J.Z. Sadler, G. Stanghellini, and T. Thornton, pp. 865–888. Oxford: Oxford University Press.

Flanagan, Owen. 2013b. The Shame of Addiction. *Frontiers in Psychiatry* 4(120), 1–11. www.frontiersin.org/articles/10.3389/fpsyt.2013.00120.

Graham, George. 2013. *The Disordered Mind: An Introduction to Philosophy of Mind and Mental Illness.* New York: Routledge.

Heather, N., M. Field, A. Moss, and S. Satel (Eds). 2022. *Evaluating the Brain Disease Model of Addiction.* New York: Routledge.

Hyman, Steven E. 1996. Addiction to Cocaine and Amphetamine. *Neuron* 16(5), 901–904. doi:10.1016/S0896-6273(00)80111-7.

Hyman, Steven E. 2007. The Neurobiology of Addiction: Implications for Voluntary Control of Behavior. *The American Journal of Bioethics* 7(1), 8–11. doi:10.1080/15265160601063969.

Holpuch, A. 2017. Route to Recovery: How People Overcome an Opioid Addiction. *The Guardian*, June 22.www.theguardian.com/us-news/2017/jun/22/opioid-addiction-america-solutions-that-work.

Jozaghi, Ehsan. 2014. 'SALOME gave my dignity back': The Role of Randomized Heroin Trials in Transforming Lives in the Downtown Eastside of Vancouver, Canada. *International Journal of Qualitative Studies in Health and Well-Being* 13 (9). doi:10.3402%2Fqhw.v9.23698.

Jopling, David A. 2000. *Self-Knowledge and the Self.* New York: Routledge.

Knapp, Caroline. 1996. *Drinking: A Love Story.* New York: Random House Publishing Group.

Kozak, Michael J. and Bruce N. Cuthbert. 2016. The NIMH Research Domain Criteria Initiative: Background, Issues, and Pragmatics. *Psychophysiology* 53(3), 286–297. doi:10.1111/psyp.12518.

Langeland, Willie, Nel Draijer, and Wim van den Brink. 2002. Trauma and Dissociation in Treatment-Seeking Alcoholics: Towards a Resolution of Inconsistent Findings." *Comprehensive Psychiatry* 43(3), 195–203. doi:10.1053/comp.2002.32350.

Leshner, Alan I. 1997. Addiction Is a Brain Disease, and It Matters. *Science* 278 (5335), 45–47. doi:10.1126/science.278.5335.45.

Machery, E. 2017. *Philosophy Within its Proper Bounds.* Oxford: Oxford University Press.

Marcenko, Maureen O., Susan P. Kemp, and Nancy C. Larson. 2000. Childhood Experiences of Abuse, Later Substance Use, and Parenting Outcomes Among Low-Income Mothers." *American Journal of Orthopsychiatry* 70(3), 316–326. doi:10.1037/h0087853.

Max, D.T. 2013. *Every Love Story is a Ghost Story: A Life of David Foster Wallace.* New York: Penguin Group.

National Center for Health Statistics. 2024. US Overdose Deaths Decrease in 2023, First Time Since 2018. Centers for Disease Control. www.cdc.gov/nchs/pressroom/nchs_press_releases/2024/20240515.htm.

Ortiz, Jordi, Lawrence W.Fitzgerald, Maura Charlton, Sarah Lane, Louis Trevisan, Xavier Guitart, William Shoemaker, Ronald S. Duman, and Eric J.Nestter. 1995. Biochemical Actions of Chronic Ethanol Exposure in the Mesolimbic Dopamine System. *Synapse* 21(4), 289–298. doi:10.1002/syn.890210403.

Oviedo-Joekes, Eugenia, Daphne Guh, Suzanne Brissette, Kristen Marchand, Scott MacDonald, Kurt Lock, Scott Harrison, et al. 2016. Hydromorphone Compared

With Diacetylmorphine for Long-Term Opioid Dependence: A Randomized Clinical Trial. *JAMA Psychiatry* 73(5), 447–455. doi:10.1001/jamapsychiatry.2016.0109.

Oviedo-Joekes, Eugenia, Bohdan Nosyk, Suzanne Brissette, Jill Chettiar, Pascal Schneeberger, David C. Marsh, Michael Krausz, Aslam Anis, and Martin T. Schechter. 2008. The North American Opiate Medication Initiative (NAOMI): Profile of Participants in North America's First Trial of Heroin-Assisted Treatment. *Journal of Urban Health* 85(6), 812–825.

Pickard, Hanna. 2021. Addiction and the Self. *Noûs* 55, 737–761.

Pickard, Hanna and Serge H. Ahmed (Eds). 2018. *The Routledge Handbook of Philosophy and Science of Addiction.* Abingdon: Routledge.

Rezapour, Tara, Parnian Rafei, Alex Baldacchino, Patricia J. Conrod, Geert Dom, Diana H. Fishbein, Atefeh Kazemi, et al. 2024. Neuroscience-Informed Classification of Prevention Interventions in Substance Use Disorders: An RDoC-Based Approach. *Neuroscience & Biobehavioral Reviews* 159, 105578. doi:10.1016/j.neubiorev.2024.105578.

Salamone, J.D., M. Correa, S.M. Mingote, and S.M. Weber. 2005. Beyond the Reward Hypothesis: Alternative Functions of Nucleus Accumbens Dopamine. *Current Opinion in Pharmacology* 5(1), 34–41. doi:10.1016/j.coph.2004.09.004.

Salamone, John D. and Mercè Correa. 2012. The Mysterious Motivational Functions of Mesolimbic Dopamine. *Neuron* 76(3), 470–485. doi:10.1016/j.neuron.2012.10.021.

Schultz, Wolfram. 2016. Dopamine Reward Prediction-Error Signalling: A Two-Component Response. *Nature Reviews Neuroscience* 17(3), 183–195. doi:10.1038/nrn.2015.26.

Steel, Daniel and Şerife Tekin. 2021. Can Treatment for Substance Use Disorder Prescribe the Same Substance as That Used? The Case of Injectable Opioid Agonist Treatment. *Kennedy Institute of Ethics Journal* 31(3), 271–301. doi:10.1353/ken.2021.0022.

Strang, John, Teodora Groshkova, Ambros Uchtenhagen, Wim van der Brink, Christian Haasen, Martin T. Schechter, Nick Lintzeris, et al. 2015. Heroin on Trial: Systematic Review and Meta-Analysis of Randomised Trials of Diamorphine-Prescribing as Treatment for Refractory Heroin Addiction. *The British Journal of Psychiatry* 207(1), 5–14. doi:10.1192/bjp.bp.114.149195.

Strevens, M. 2019. *Thinking off Your Feet: How Empirical Psychology Vindicates Armchair Philosophy.* Cambridge, MA: Harvard University Press.

Supporters of SALOME. 2017. To Whom it May Concern': Dispatches from SALOME and The Crosstown Clinic.

Tabb, Kathryn. 2017. On the Ethics of Precision: Funding Priorities and Diachronic Justice in Psychiatry. Master's Thesis. University of Pittsburgh.

Tabb, Kathryn. 2020. Should Psychiatry be Precise? Reduction, Big Data, and Nosological Revision in Mental Health Research. In *Levels of Analysis in Psychopathology*, edited by Kenneth K. Kendler, Josef Parnas, and Peter Zachar, pp. 308–334. Cambridge: Cambridge University Press.

Tabb, Kathryn. 2023. Precision. In *Keywords for Health Humanities*, edited by Sari Altschuler, JonathanMetzl, and Priscilla Wald, pp. 167–170. Cambridge, MA: MIT Press.

Tanz, Lauren J, Amanda T. Dinwiddie, Stephanie Snodgrass, Julie O'Donnell, Christine L. Mattson, and Nicole L. Davis. 2022. A Qualitative Assessment of Circumstances Surrounding Drug Overdose Deaths During the Early Stages of the COVID-19 Pandemic. SUDORS Data Brief 2. Centers for Disease Control and Prevention.

Tekin, Şerife. 2011. Self-Concept through the Diagnostic Looking Glass: Narratives and Mental Disorder. *Philosophical Psychology* 24(3), 357–380. doi:10.1080/09515089.2011.559622.

Tekin, Şerife. 2014a. The Missing Self in Hacking's Looping Effects. In *Classifying Psychopathology: Mental Kinds and Natural Kinds*, edited by H. Kincaid and J.A. Sullivan, pp. 227–256. Cambridge, MA: Boston Review. doi:10.7551/mitpress/8942.001.0001.

Tekin, Şerife. 2014b. Self-Insight in the Time of Mood Disorders: After the Diagnosis, Beyond the Treatment. *Philosophy, Psychiatry, & Psychology* 21(4), 139–144. doi:10.1353/ppp.2014.0019.

Tekin, Şerife. 2014c. A Perfect Storm: Health, Disorder, Culture, and the Self. *Philosophy, Psychiatry, & Psychology* 21(2), 165–168. doi:10.1353/ppp.2014.0024.

Tekin, Şerife. 2015. Against Hyponarrating Grief: Incompatible Research and Treatment Interests in the DSM-5. In *The DSM-5 in Perspective*, edited by Steeves Demazeux and Patrick Singy, pp. 179–197. Dordrecht: Springer Netherlands. doi:10.1007/978-94-017-9765-8_11.

Tekin, Şerife. 2021. Self and Mental Disorder: Lessons for Psychiatry from Naturalistic Philosophy. *Philosophy Compass* 16(1), e12715. doi:10.1111/phc3.12715.

Tekin, Şerife. 2023. Philosophy of Psychiatry Meets Experimental Philosophy: Expertise Naturalized. In *Advances in Experimental Philosophy of Medicine*, edited by Kristien Hens and Andreas De Block, pp. 305–321. London: Bloomsbury Academic.

Tekin, Şerife, Alicia A. Swan, Willie J. Hale, and Mary Jo Pugh. 2022. Understanding Substance Use Disorders among Veterans: Virtues of the Multitudinous Self Model. In *Evaluating the Brain Disease Model of Addiction*, edited by Nick Heather, Matt Field, Anthony Moss, and Sally Satel. London: Routledge.

Volkow, Nora D. 2018. What Does It Mean When We Call Addiction a Brain Disorder?. *Scientific American Blog Network*. https://blogs.scientificamerican.com/observations/what-does-it-mean-when-we-call-addiction-a-brain-disorder.

Volkow, Nora D., George F. Koob, and A. Thomas McLellan. 2016. Neurobiologic Advances from the Brain Disease Model of Addiction. *New England Journal of Medicine* 374(4), 363–371. doi:10.1056/NEJMra1511480.

West, Robert and Jamie Brown. 2013. *Theory of Addiction*. Chichester: John Wiley & Sons.

World Health Organization, United Nations Office on Drugs and Crimes, UNAIDS. 2004. Substitution Maintenance Therapy in the Management of Opioid Dependence and HIV/AIDS Prevention. www.who.int/publications/i/item/who-unodc-unaids-position-paper.-substitution-maintenance-therapy-in-the-management-of-opioid-dependence-and-hiv-aids-prevention.

Epilogue

In *Labyrinths*, Borges writes that every writer creates their own precursors and their work "modifies our conception of the past, as it will modify the future" (Borges 1962). I hope *Reclaiming the Self in Psychiatry: Centering Personal Narratives for a Humanist Science* fulfills Borges's prophecy. My project, as I wrote at the start, was to pay attention to what individuals with mental disorders had to say about their experiences, so that I could identify the shortcomings of contemporary scientific approaches to mental disorders and offer a way to address them. After a deep engagement with the self-narratives of patients and a historical and philosophical reading of psychiatry's past, with a focus on its efforts to establish itself as simultaneously a discipline of science and medical care, I identified psychiatry's sidestepping of the self as the main culprit. In doing so, I gestured to a future in which the self, in its full complexity and richness, is at the center of attending to individuals' encounters with mental distresses and disorders.

Psychiatry's commitment to scientifically unpack the nature of mental disorder by turning to its easily measurable constituents, such as clusters of behavior or faulty brain chemistry, has resulted in the downplaying of the psychological, social, cultural, and linguistic complexity of the self who is the subject of mental disorders. Patients' experiences and testimonies are not part of psychiatric knowledge, and the concept of the self is not studied in psychiatry as it is in cognitive sciences and philosophy. Although describing mental disorders in terms of behavior or physical mechanisms isolated from the overall complexity of the person who encounters them has yielded improved scientific explanations, it has inadvertently created a framework for mental disorders that is not fully responsive to the needs of individuals. By engaging with both historical and philosophical insights and the first-person reports of those who have mental distresses and disorders, I showed how overlooking the self in psychiatry has had epistemic and ethical costs, first, in the context of the clinical interventions that aim to help patients flourish, and second, in the context of individuals' reflections about themselves and the narratives they create to make sense of and respond to their mental distresses and disorders. I proposed the Multitudinous Self Model (*MuSe*) as a way to reduce these costs.

DOI: 10.4324/9781003055556-11

MuSe integrates three bodies of information to display the complexity of the self and provide conceptual and empirical tools for responding to mental distresses and disorders. The sources of information I used to develop *MuSe* reflect my own training and interests as an empirically oriented philosopher for whom philosophical thinking is useful not just for decomposition but also for synthesis and integration. *MuSe* relies on 1) first-person reports or testimonies of those diagnosed with mental disorders; 2) empirical research on the self, grounded in the cognitive and behavioral sciences and thus reflecting the significance of biological, cognitive, social, and cultural factors shaping the encounter with mental distresses and disorders; and 3) philosophical approaches to the self posited by empirically informed philosophers.

My invitation to scientifically investigate, clinically intervene in, and personally make sense of mental disorders through *MuSe* has two goals. The first can be encapsulated as remedial work: *MuSe* has conceptual and empirical resources to address and remedy the epistemic and ethical costs of underappreciating the self in psychiatry. It does so by conceptualizing what it means to have a mental disorder, making a pragmatic distinction between mental distress and mental disorder. Such a distinction situates mental distresses and disorders on the broad continuum of human cognitive diversity and opens up resources for individuals to receive the (sometimes medical) interventions necessary for flourishing without necessarily categorizing their complex experiences under a diagnostic label or doing so only in certain contexts when it provides useful resources. The second goal can be encapsulated as enlargement work: *MuSe* provides additional conceptual and empirical tools for psychiatry to aid flourishing by integrating first-person testimonies, research in cognitive sciences, and empirically informed philosophy. In addition, *MuSe* improves psychiatry's relationship with science by promoting more expansive and sophisticated notions of expertise and objectivity.

It is my hope that *MuSe* will serve as a source of inspiration and motivation for scientists, clinicians, clinical trainees, educators, policymakers, and patients to rethink how to reflect on, study, learn about, and manage mental disorders and develop self-friendly frameworks to respond to experiences of mental distresses and disorders. I envision *MuSe* as an interface, a bridge, a connection between the more systematized and scientific strands of psychiatry, the art, skill, and technical expertise of the clinicians who treat patients, and the experience-based expertise of individuals who encounter mental distresses and disorders and have much to say about what helps or impedes their flourishing. *MuSe* places philosophy at the center of reflecting on mental disorders, both as an analytic discipline that offers critical thinking tools for a meta-analysis of the states of affairs in scientific, clinical, cultural, and personal contexts in which mental distresses and disorders are experienced and examined, and as a practical activity able to explore and explain rich concepts such as autonomy, agency, flourishing, and a good life.

Reclaiming the Self in Psychiatry: Centering Personal Narratives for a Humanist Science has made a start in this direction, but more remains to be done. By putting the self at the center of thinking about what it means for individuals to have mental distresses and disorders, psychiatry can benefit from the rich philosophical literature and the wisdom of individuals who want to make their lives better.

Finally, embracing the rich diversity of persons—of selves—as a starting point when responding to mental distresses and disorders will nurture values of curiosity, humility, tolerance, compassion, and respect, resulting in an appreciation of the many different kinds of minds and respect for their unique paths to excellence and flourishing.

References

Borges, Jorge Luis. 1962. *Labyrinths*. Translated by James E. Irby, Donald A. Yates, John M. Fein, Harriet de Onís, Julian Palley, Dudley Fitts, and L.A. Murillo. New York: New Directions Publishing Corporation.

Index

Printed in the United States
by Baker & Taylor Publisher Services